Community Care for Health Professionals

Community Care for Health Professionals

Edited by

Ann Compton MSCP, Grad Dip Phys, SRP
Practising Community Physiotherapist; formerly Course Tutor, Diploma in Community Physiotherapy, Southampton Institute of Higher Education, Southampton, UK

Mary Ashwin BA, Dip Soc Admin, AIMSW, Cert Ed, MPhil
Senior Lecturer in Applied Social Studies, Southampton Institute of Higher Education, Southampton, UK

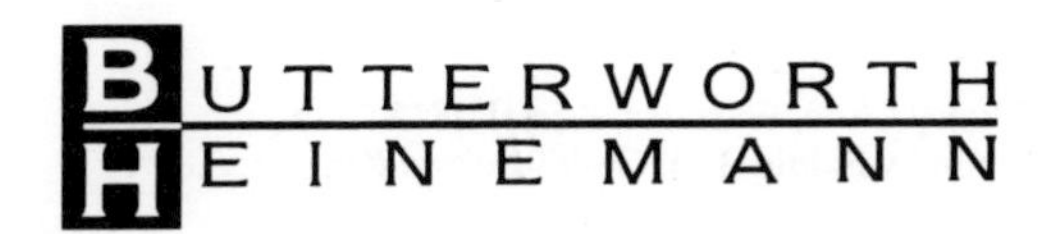

Butterworth-Heinemann Ltd
Linacre House, Jordan Hill, Oxford OX2 8DP

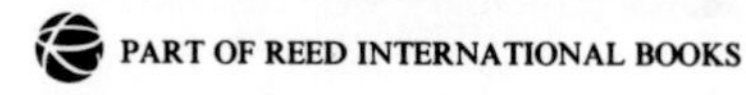

OXFORD LONDON BOSTON
MUNICH NEW DELHI SINGAPORE SYDNEY
TOKYO TORONTO WELLINGTON

First published 1992

British Library Cataloguing in Publication Data
Community Care for Health
Professionals
I. Compton, Ann II. Ashwin, Mary
361.8

ISBN 0 7506 0185 X

Typeset by BC Typesetting, 23 Exley Close, Warmley, Bristol BS15 5YD
Printed and bound in Great Britain by Biddles Ltd, Guildford and King's Lynn

Contents

Contributors

Tony Acland BSc, MA
Principal Lecturer in Sociology and Deputy Head of the Social Science Division at Southampton Institute of Higher Education. He is an experienced lecturer in sociology having taught the subject to community nurses, physiotherapista nd other health professionals for many years.

Mary Ashwin BA, Dip Soc Admin, AIMSW, Cert Ed, MPhil
Senior Lecturer in Applied Social Studies at Southampton Institute of Higher Education. Her background is in medical social work and child care. She is an experienced teacher, having taught a wide range of practitioners in the caring professions. She works as a counsellor and has a special interest in the care of the elderly.

Ron Chalk MSc, BEd, CQSW
Principal Lecturer in Applied Social Studies at Southampton Institute of Higher Education. He trained originally in youth and community work but moved to social work at the time of the Seebohm reorganisation. He has been actively involved in group and community work and training since the mid-1970s.

Ann Compton MSCP, Grad Dip Phys, SRP
A practising community physiotherapist with many years experience, she was until recently Course Coordinator for the Diploma in Community Physiotherapy at Southampton Institute. Founder chairperson and newsletter editor of the Association of Community Physiotherapists (a specific interest group of the Chartered Society of Physiotherapy), she also piloted the Introduction and Orientation to Community Physiotherapy course, and has lectured widely and written on community-based physiotherapy practice.

Howard Davis BA, LlB, PhD
Principal Lecturer in Law and Leader of the Law Section in the Business Division at the Southampton Institute of Higher Education. His teaching and research spans both public and private law.

He has considerable experience in the education of mature students and the production of learning materials to meet the needs of those in full-time work.

Sandra Horn CPsychol, BTech (Hons Psych), Dip Clin Psych
Clinical Psychologist and Lecturer on MSc in Rehabilitation Studies course at the University of Southampton. She has written a number of self-help books on topics such as managing stress, pain relief without drugs and coping with bereavement.

Val Jones BA, Cert Ed, CQSW
Senior Lecturer in Applied Social Studies at Southampton Institute of Higher Education. She has a background in residential and field social work, primarily with children and families. Her current interests include family work, counselling and issues of consumer involvement.

Derek Williams BSc, Cert Ed, MSc
Senior Lecturer in Sociology and Social Policy at Southampton Institute of Higher Education. He has taught widely on professional and degree courses and in further education. He is a member of the Association for the Teaching of Social Sciences and also the Policy Studies Association.

Preface

This book is designed for health professionals and gives the necessary additional knowledge and skills needed to adapt from institutional to community-based care. It focuses upon those aspects of community practice which are common to all workers and adopts a holistic approach in which respect for service users is central. It assumes that the practitioner will be equipped with his or her own specific professional expertise.

Key aspects of social policy, sociology and psychology, together with legal issues, are addressed clearly and concisely. They are set alongside the necessary additional skills for successful community practice. Throughout the book case material and practical exercises allow readers to develop their own knowledge and expertise. Developed from the Diploma in Community Physiotherapy, this handbook will be of value to all health professionals working in the community or preparing to do so.

Acknowledgements

This book would not have been written without the five years of stimulation and critical feedback from the Diploma in Community Physiotherapy students at Southampton Institute.

Ann Compton and Mary Ashwin would also wish to thank their families: John, Paul, Maggie, Sarah and John, for their advice, tolerance and practical assistance; Timmy, Horry, Harrie and Timmy for their companionship and forbearance.

Introduction

The aim of the book

This book is about the knowledge and skills required by community practitioners such as physiotherapists working outside institutional settings in what is somewhat loosely called 'the community'. Its aim is to provide information and technical know-how essential for a community-based practitioner.

The content

The book has been divided into two main sections. The first looks at what the community practitioner needs to know; the second identifies the necessary skills required to deliver an effective service. Examples and practice exercises are offered throughout.

The knowledge base

The aim of this section is to enable the practitioner to practise in an informed, sensitive and intelligent way.

Social context

This examines the social policies which determine both the nature and level of provision as well as the legal framework on which this provision is based (Chapters 2, 3 and 4).

Psychology

The community practitioner also requires an appreciation of the individual's behaviour and the needs and drives which fuel it. This section will focus on areas of common concern: ageing, sexuality, pain, grief and common adjustments to disability (Chapter 5).

The skills base

This is concerned with common areas of practice with which the practitioner may be familiar but where skill development is crucial. It describes the skills involved and provides exercises for their practice which together raise important questions about their relevance, application and implementation.

Working with individuals

This section promotes the development of the necessary skills for effective communication in one to one situations (Chapter 6).

The helping process

This identifies the core skills required by the community practitioner, which are assessment, programme planning and evaluation (Chapter 7).

Working with families

The community practitioner is made aware of the importance of family systems and equipped with some basic skills to work within the family setting (Chapter 8).

Working with groups

It can be more economical and effective for the practitioner to work with groups. This chapter describes some strategies which will develop good working practice (Chapter 9).

Working in the community

This chapter looks at factors which affect service delivery and their influences upon the practitioner's delivery of care (Chapter 10).

Teaching in the community

Teaching is a skill which has relevance to many aspects of community work. This chapter gives practical advice to both teachers and supervisors (Chapter 11).

Concluding exercises

Outlines of some cases by which practitioners can test out their working knowledge are included.

The presentation

A major consideration throughout the planning and writing of this book has been that the information it contains should be readily accessible to the busy community practitioner. It was also a major concern that the need for clarity and brevity should not conflict with the demands of accuracy and comprehensiveness.

Each chapter serves as an introduction to the topics, all of which are of great importance. Exercises are included to enable the practitioner to relate the information more readily to their own practice. Additional sources of information are also indicated when appropriate. In this way the book may be used to highlight areas of need and provide a good basis from which to undertake further study.

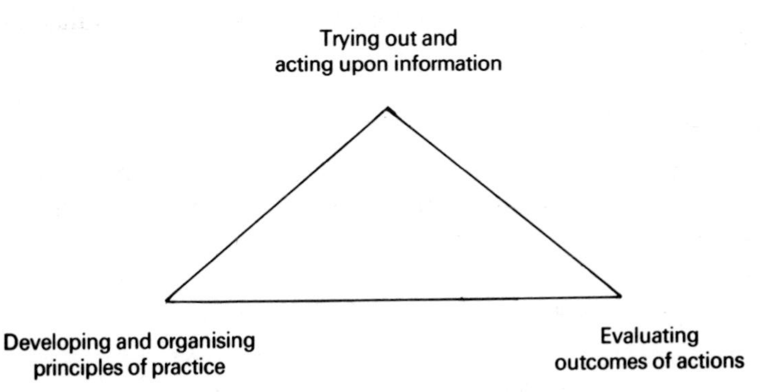

Part One

Essential Knowledge Base

Chapter 1

An introduction to community care

Mary Ashwin and Ann Compton

1. The origin

The concept of community care is as vague as its current usage. As early as 1961 Professor Richard Titmus was mystified as to its origin. Its first appearance in official documents was in the report of the Royal Commission on Mental Illness and Mental Deficiency 1957. It was used from then on increasingly, not always to describe the same thing, but usually directed towards the care of certain groups. The main recipients of this care were people suffering from mental illness, those experiencing learning difficulties or the frail elderly population. The two main groups of professionals involved in providing this care were Health and Social Service workers.

2. Definitions

Community care has been variously defined. In the earlier reports it was used to identify any care given outside large institutions, including that within smaller locally based residential establishments, such as Cheshire Homes and 46 bedded homes for the elderly.

Gradually this has now changed so that it now

- excludes most residential establishments of any size used on a permanent basis;
- includes both statutory and voluntary services as well as personal social networks with special emphasis on family care.

3. Distinctions

Two useful distinctions were highlighted by Martin Bulmer (1987). He draws attention to the difference between care 'IN' the community and care 'BY' the community.

- Care 'IN' the community includes care in locally based institutions and domiciliary care provided by a range of paid staff.
- Care 'BY' the community is seen as referring to care by family, friends and local voluntary bodies.

He sees the trend in official policy increasingly towards this form of care.

The second distinction between FORMAL and INFORMAL carers is harder to define. It covers the whole range of services from formal statutory care through commercially provided care and voluntary care to informal care (Chapter 2). All these types of care are seen as interdependent though the precise nature of their enmeshing is complex.

4. Targeting

The target of community care has also changed over time. The Seebohm Report (1968) saw community care as a re-integrative process for those who had become isolated or disaffected. It now tends to be defined as a policy which seeks to provide supportive services from a range of sources in order to provide the user with a situation as close to 'normal' everyday life as possible. Clearly words such as 'normal' are open to a multitude of interpretations but in the 1989 White Paper it was linked to 'care packages for individuals', thus somewhat faintly echoing the Griffiths concern for 'client choice'.

The sort of care provided to achieve this current goal will consist of a mixture of physical caring and psychological and environmental support. The distribution of these tasks between the informal and formal carers is seen as negotiable.

5. Service delivery

The community practitioner faces a formidable challenge; she or he is required to undertake a task with an infinitely variable range of collaborations. The only common clear objective is the rather negative one of avoiding institutionalisation.

Exercise

Write a description of community care as it might appear to a:

(a) civil servant;

(b) colleague;
(c) service user;
(d) family carer.

What are the main conflicts highlighted in the different descriptions?

The development of community based practice – a case example

With the inception of the National Health Service (NHS) in 1948, health care was divided into three service areas: hospital, family practitioner and community.

Community health services were mainly the province of the Health Department of a County, Borough or City Council. These included all environmental health services, maternal and child welfare, health visiting, home nursing services, vaccination and immunisation, and the care and after-care of mentally ill and mentally handicapped people. Some of these services had been provided by voluntary agencies, and these were either absorbed into the NHS or provided with financial help. School medical services were run in conjunction with the Council's Education Department. Industrial health services were organised by the Ministry of Labour via the Factory Inspectorate, whilst the Armed services retained their own health services separate from the NHS.

Physiotherapy was seen as a scarce resource. Its main provision under the NHS was restricted to hospitals, except in Scotland where the nature of the scattered population made it desirable to maintain orthopaedic aftercare. Variations in the rest of the UK included:

- Some areas had charitably funded mobile physiotherapy services which did not attract NHS funding. Some were closed but others were maintained by voluntary contributions and fundraising.
- Some physiotherapists with their own practices chose to become private practitioners rather than be absorbed into the NHS.
- A few industries employed physiotherapists.
- A relatively small number of physiotherapists were employed by education authorities, usually for 'delicate' children.

At that time physiotherapy could only be prescribed by a medical practitioner.

Within the NHS most general practitioners only had access to the hospital-based treatments through referral to a hospital-based practitioner. This meant that the majority of patients had to see a hospital consultant before they were able to receive physiotherapy. This often involved a long delay between problem identification and treatment.

This situation remained virtually unchanged despite medical and professional developments until 1971 when professional concerns and Government events coincided.

A number of practice issues emerged:

- Physiotherapists were realising the value of pre-discharge home visits for patients with major disabilities. Rehabilitation programmes could then be tailored more realistically to lifestyle.
- When carers were invited to attend departments they were taught essential techniques for caring safely, but because there were major discrepancies between the home and institutional environment only some of the problems were ameliorated.
- Physiotherapists were also concerned that there was no provision for those patients who needed or were prescribed therapy but were too debilitated, or exhausted by travel, to attend outpatient appointments.
- Other patients regularly returned for courses of treatment, stating they could not manage at home without some support. Often there was little that the therapist could offer clinically.
- Frequently patients with acute conditions were having to wait, often several months, to be seen by consultants. These acute conditions could have been relieved instead of developing into chronic problems with subsequent damaging effects upon the patients' social, economic and psychological welfare.

In 1970 two Acts of Parliament came into effect:

□ the Education (Handicapped Children) Act.
□ the Chronically Sick and Disabled Persons' Act.

Both had clauses within them that enabled local authorities to make provisions for needs they identified. This created an opportunity for the appointment of physiotherapists by Education, Health or Social Services departments.

It was upon this rather insubstantial legal base that community physiotherapy was established. There emerged a number of differences between hospital and community practice. In the community:

□ little equipment was used;
□ patients and carers were taught long-term management within their own environment;

- practice became based on the individual's needs within the family and wider social context.

The community physiotherapist's role altered from that of a 'specialist' within a relatively narrow field to that of a community-based health practitioner. To meet this new challenge the traditional knowledge and skills base needed expansion. Examples would include:

- knowledge of preventative health measures and health promotion to respond to individual, family and community issues;
- knowledge of national and local social, educational and voluntary services;
- knowledge of the legal framework for community practice;
- in the absence of a common institutional culture, an ability to demonstrate respect for each individual's lifestyle, attitudes and beliefs;
- a knowledge of a different and more complex range of personal and organisational management issues.

The Health Service reorganisation of 1974 resulted in the transfer of the community health services, with the exemption of environmental health, from Local Authorities to the National Health Service. Existing community physiotherapy services became integrated with the District Physiotherapy Service. From isolated local initiatives community physiotherapy quickly became a recognised component of District Health policies.

As the task was more complex and the physiotherapist found herself working in relative isolation from the mutually supportive environment of a hospital the Association of Community Physiotherapists was formed (1980). This is a specific interest group of the Chartered Society of Physiotherapy whose aims include education and mutual support. This was a recognition that there was a difference between institutional and community based practice.

Exercise

Trace the evolution of your own community service.

References

Bulmer, M. (1987) *The Social Basis of Community Care*. London: Allen & Unwin.

NIMH (1961) Report of the Annual Conference of The National Association for Mental Health, speech by Professor R. M. Titmus, reproduced in R M Titmus (1968) *Commitment to Welfare*. London: Allen & Unwin, Chapter ix.

Report of the Royal Commission on Mental Illness and Mental Deficiency (1957) (cmnd 169). London: HMSO.

Seebohm Report (1968) *Report of the Committee on Local Authority and Allied Personal Social Services* (cmnd 3703). London: HMSO.

White Paper (1989) *Caring for People: Community Care in the Next Decade and Beyond* (cmnd 849). London: HMSO.

Further reading

Brown, M. and Payne, S. (1990) *Introduction to Social Administration in Britain.* London: Unwin Hyman.

Byrne, T. and Padfield, C. F. (1985) *Social Services Made Simple.* London: Heinemann.

Clark, J. and Henderson, J. (1983) *Community Health.* Edinburgh: Churchill Livingstone.

Jones, K. (1989) Community care: old problems and new answers. In Carter, P., Jeffs, T. and Smith, M. (eds) *Social Work and Social Welfare. Yearbook I.* Milton Keynes: Open University Press.

Langan, M. (1990) Community care in the 1990s: the community care White Paper 'Caring for People'. In *Critical Social Policy*, Autumn 1990.

Ottewill, R. and Wall, A. (1990) *Community Health Services.* London: Business Education Publishers Ltd.

Chapter 2

Social policy and provision

Derek Williams

Introduction

The issue of community care is one to which analysts of social policy have paid a good deal of attention through the last decade. This has happened for a whole variety of reasons, but perhaps the main one is that the issue is one which highlights an age-old dichotomy within policy analysis – that of policy formulation and implementation. The thinking underlying this dichotomy is that there exists a gap, or 'deficit', between the intentions of policy-makers (politicians and civil servants), and the reality of practice, 'at the coalface' within most, if not all, policy areas (Ham and Hill 1984, pp. 95, 96).

This gap between policy and practice has led some to question the notion that any clear distinction can be made between the two activities, and that the problem would be better reformulated as a continuum, rather than a process consisting of discrete phases (Barrat and Fudge 1981). For community practitioners and social scientists in general, these questions are of interest since their attention is often focused on the unintentional consequences of human action (Giddens 1989). For them, the existence of an 'implementation deficit' is a normal feature of social reality, whereas for policy-makers, looking from the top, down towards the area of practice, any such deficit is viewed as a problem to be solved.

Policy-makers themselves, of course, are not unaware that policy statements and policy guidelines often fail to effectively bring about the desired outcomes. Sir Roy Griffiths recognised this problem in the area of community care:

> Community care has been talked of for 30 years, and in few areas can the gap between political rhetoric and policy on one hand, or between policy and reality in the field on the other hand have been so great (Griffiths 1988).

The aim of this chapter is to document the historical development of community care policy during the post-war period. It also aims to analyse that development and the current policy position, within a framework which focuses on the issue of implementation. This should enable the reader to understand the evolution of the policy and to analyse some of the issues surrounding the current policy debate.

Key concepts

Implementation problems may arise if confusion or ambiguity exists over key *concepts* within the policy statements. The policy of community care rests, as is obvious, on the concepts of 'community' and 'care', both of which have been seen as problematic and open to misreading and misunderstanding. The notion of a community implies an idea of mutual support, trust and, above all, a degree of altruism. As Professor Halsey has recently suggested, these ideas are not congruent with any kind of contractual service, or with market forces (Halsey 1990). Janet Finch has raised similar doubts about the concept of community and argues that it is a mythical construction which serves to deflect attention away from the State's responsibility towards vulnerable groups in society (Finch 1982).

Similar ambiguity surrounds the concept of 'care'. It is a concept which, when 'unpacked', reveals a range of meanings. Roy Parker (1981) suggests that its central meaning is better described as 'tending', that is, paying close attention to the physical needs of the person as well as their emotional and psychological needs. This is not necessarily the equivalent of 'caring about' someone, implying a capacity for empathy and emotional involvement. In the professionalisation of care, objectives of efficiency and a concern for effective time-management may conflict with notions of empathy since the latter can involve a sense of timeless commitment for the person being 'cared for'. Carers themselves have sometimes described the texture of caring and the need to spend time.

'Patients can ask for a lot from you. You have to really listen to them. Listen to them, it will do them some good. People sit in a chair here all day, waiting for someone to just talk to them, to wash them, to give them their food' (Glouberman 1991).

The activity of caring then is perhaps misrepresented by the word 'care' as used in the concept of community care. Moreover, these activities are particularly crucial in the lives of many women. Finch (1982) has argued that policy statements and political rhetoric concerning care hide the facts about women's primary involvement in caring for others; not only young children, but also elderly, sick and disabled relatives. During the period since the 1950s this caring has increasingly been combined with women's involvement in paid employment.

The activity of caring then, upon closer inspection reveals aspects other than simply altruism. As Mary Langan points out, the logic of those proposals contained within the Government's White Paper on Community Care which emphasise the need for a 'mixed economy of care' and some degree of reliance on the private sector, has a negative impact on care workers since 'cost-effectiveness' is achieved by reducing their pay, hours and conditions of work. Such utilitarian approaches sit uneasily with our usual notions of care (Langan 1990).

The evolution of the policy

1. The 1950s and 1960s

It is important now to trace the evolution of community care policies in the post-war period, since the present policies have their origins in many of the debates and changes which occurred through the 1960s and 1970s. It was the Royal Commission on the Law Relating to Mental Illness and Mental Deficiency (1954–1957) which first coined the term 'community care', and, as others have pointed out, the Ministry of Health advocated domiciliary services for the elderly in 1958 (Open University 1984, p. 93). The new stress on 'informal patients', contained in the 1959 Mental Health Act – 'who could come or go without detention or certification', reflected a general questioning of the effectiveness of institutional care and an emphasis on control of the patient.

The critique of carceral forms of care and control was a powerful theme in the sociological literature of the 1960s, notably in the writings of Erving Goffman. Goffman's book, *Asylums*, carefully analysed the features of 'total institutions' – prisons, hospitals, monasteries and the like and pointed up the negative consequences for 'inmates'. Such institutions, particularly if of a coercive nature, will have the effect of depersonalising the individual and systematically eroding their social identity (Goffman 1961).

Goffman's writings coincided with a general shift in emphasis away from the large, custodial institution, towards more localised, small-scale provision of NHS hospitals (Open University 1984). Thus, academic analysis and policy shifts worked together to bring about a changing climate of opinion. Official thinking reflected this and official documents spoke openly of community care. The White Paper 'Health and Welfare: the Development of Community Care'

(Ministry of Health 1966) talked in terms of domiciliary staff, health centres and clinics as being prerequisites for community care provision.

This period in the early to mid-1960s witnessed the *conception* and *formulation* of the policy. The task of translating these ideas into a practical community care policy has proved to be very difficult, and this has been recognised by many commentators (Jaehnig 1979, p. 3).

This has been partly due to the lack of clarity mentioned earlier, but inadequate planning and resources must be seen as largely responsible. Those who suffered most were the mentally ill and the mentally handicapped. As Langan points out (1990), the mentally ill were often discharged into the care of relatives who were provided with little additional support. Many of the mentally handicapped remained confined to long-stay institutions. Mental handicap throughout the post-war period held the status of a 'cinderella' service and resources for community care for this client group remained a low priority. Despite the fact that the period after 1968 and the publication of the Seebohm Report on local authority Social Services, a steady increase in funding (Seebohm 1968) was witnessed. As Neil Evans has recently pointed out, Social Services Departments' expenditure increased by 68% between 1968 and 1973 (Evans 1990). The move towards de-institutionalisation of the mentally handicapped continued and the 1971 document, 'Better Services for the Mentally Handicapped' (DHSS 1971), recommended that hospitals no longer be used for residential care; rather local authorities would be the providers of residential accommodation and a variety of forms of care would be developed with the support of the social work profession. There is an optimism prevalent which arises out of the absence of doubts about the continuing flow of resources and a vision of social work practice as being capable of tackling (and solving!) a wide range of care problems.

By the time of publication of the companion White Paper, 'Better Services for the Mentally Ill' (DHSS 1975) there was perhaps, less optimism. As Alan Walker has pointed out, the policy was reaffirmed but no strategy was proposed to implement the closure of large psychiatric hospitals (Walker 1982).

2. The 1970s

The 1970s, and particularly the latter half of the decade, saw a good deal of policy debate directed towards considerations of 'normalisation' and 'integration'. The former concept (which lay behind much of the de-institutionalisation of the period), is most closely associated with Wolfensberger (1972), and fits with notions of community care in so far as it advocates treating the mentally handicapped as ordinary citizens with full citizenship rights. The latter concept became known through the recommendations of the Warnock Report (1978). The Report proposed that, where feasible and appropriate, handicapped children should be integrated into normal schools, though this integration might take a variety of forms to be determined at the discretion of the relevant professionals. The report coined the terms 'special needs' and 'learning difficulty' which have since become more commonplace terms and are used by the majority of social service and health professionals. Changes in language of themselves, however, are relatively ineffectual and, although the Labour Government embraced Warnock, the Conservatives' 1980 White Paper and the subsequent 1981 Education Act followed its central themes, there was almost no reference to and certainly no commitment to providing the necessary resources.

3. The 1980s

Thus, by the opening of the 1980s, the main lines of policy debate, at least, had become clarified. The talk was now of non-institutional care, 'integration', 'normalisation' and 'care in the community'. The rise to prominence of these powerful and emotive symbolic words and phrases coincided with the emergence of a style of government committed to reining back public expenditure and taking a searching look at the value and cost effectiveness of services such as health and the social services. Indeed, the Conservative Government which came to office in 1979 was concerned to reappraise the whole enterprise of state-provided welfare. Welfare provision was now viewed as both an economic problem – depressing incentives and 'realistic' wage levels, and a moral problem – inhibiting individual self-reliance and undermining the centrality of the family (Evans 1990).

This ideological coincidence began to stifle any further analysis of community care policy. Genuine notions of community were hijacked by the thinkers and gurus of the 'New Right', and as they bent the ears of ministers and civil servants, by politicians themselves. In a period of anti-statism, concepts like community and family came to stand for the small-scale, the intimate, and the altruistic. It allowed social services ministers to mingle these concepts with notions like a 'mixed economy' of welfare and the value of the private sector. As Michael Bayley saw it, in 1973, the shift in emphasis was from 'care in the community', to 'care by the community' (Bayley 1973). This marked an important change in direction for the policy of community care and reflects an earlier point about the uncertain consequences of policy intention when translated into action; that is to say, the critics of institutions and the early advocates of de-institutionalisation and normalisation would barely have recognised the debates of the mid-1980s, focusing, as they did, on a style of provision 'that interweaves statutory and informal care' (Bayley 1978).

The increasing role of the non-statutory sector was an important feature of the 1980s. Pressure groups, self-help groups and others took on a more campaigning and active role. This represented a challenge to traditional, statutory forms of provision and ways of working. The White Paper 'Caring for People' formalises that local authorities should develop an increasingly contractual relationship with voluntary agencies. The White Paper, following Griffiths, states that this will serve to 'clarify the role of voluntary agencies; give them a sounder financial base . . .' and 'enhance the development of more flexible and cost-effective forms of non-statutory provision' (CM849 1989). Lunn (1989) believes, however, that contracting out services to voluntary organisations is not an appropriate area for expansion, since the majority of such organisations remain responsive to need by remaining small and local. It seems likely, too, that some of the larger national voluntary bodies will taken an increasingly critical stance towards government if adequate resources are not forthcoming for the particular client group they represent. The Spastics Society, for example, have recently been extremely vocal on the government's failure to fully implement the 1986 Disabled Persons' Act.

Making a reality of community care

The next significant landmark in the evolution of community care policy was the 1986 Audit Commission's Report, 'Making a Reality of Community Care'. The Commission, given its long-standing brief to investigate and identify inefficient use of resources, put forward a major criticism of government policy, namely, that value for money was not being achieved, despite an annual financial outlay on long-term care of some £6 billion. As Kathleen Jones has pointed out, local authorities were penalised by rate-capping and restrictions on the Public Sector Borrowing Requirement. This severely limited their efforts to build up community services (Jones 1989). Jones notes that the consequence of this squeeze on public sector services was the very rapid growth of the private sector, 'much of which was supported out of public funds'. In the early 1980s, it became possible to obtain Social Security payments to fund a stay in residential care, providing means-test criteria were met. Such subsidy costs could be as high as £200 per week, per individual, and this amounted to, in the words of the Commission, 'Policy conflicts and perverse incentives'. As was noted in the introductory remarks, policy intentions frequently result in unintended and unforeseen consequences. In its recommendations, the Audit Commission attached central importance to the role of the local manager in controlling budgets and exercising considerable discretion over the purchase of services; an important theme in subsequent debates over community care provision. A more negative, though equally unintended, consequence has been noted by Tessa Jowell of the Joseph Rowntree Foundation – namely, that the supplementary benefit (now income support) paid out to elderly people in private residential care does not always meet the full cost of their care. This gap in funding has variously been met by 'charities, on a Robin Hood Principle [cross-subsidy between residents within the same home] and on families' (Jowell 1990 – my brackets).

The dilemmas facing policy-makers had become more pointed, therefore, and it became apparent that it would be difficult in practice to combine curbs on public expenditure and a desire to encourage the private sector of welfare with effective community care. Sir Roy Griffiths, deputy Director of the Sainsbury's Supermarket chain, was appointed to formulate a succinct report to the government. Unlike many previous reports, this broke with the tradition of Royal Commissions and public enquiries, by adopting a style of straightforward fact-finding and evidence collecting, aiming to produce a set of recommendations in a short period.

The Griffiths Report

Griffiths made a number of proposals, but central was the idea, derived from the Audit Commission report, that a 'community care manager' should be able to purchase services from wherever he or she thought appropriate. This would mean the public or the private sector. Local Authority Social Service Departments were now to act in a facilitative role, as 'the designers, organisers and purchasers of non-health care services' (Griffiths 1988). This clearly would have the effect of removing their role as direct providers, but gave them a pivotal role in Planning.

The White Paper

The Government's White Paper, 'Caring for People', followed Griffiths closely, but its reception was not unproblematic. A good deal of critical debate has centred around the changed role of the local authority Social Services and the concepts of consumer choice and service flexibility. Mary Langan, for example, has argued that the actual outcome of Social Service departments becoming 'enablers' aiming for a 'mixed economy' of care is likely to be:

> a two-tier welfare system in which the private and voluntary sectors look after anybody who can raise the required funds and the local authority deals with a residuum of the poorest, the most disturbed and the most difficult (Langan 1990, p. 64).

Clearly, this is a new pattern for local authority staff which will require learning new methods of working and new ways of thinking about care provision.

The White Paper also envisages that local authority Social Service departments will provide a 'care manager' for the important activity of 'case management'. This will include:

- the identification of people in need;
- an assessment of care needs;
- the planning and securing of care delivery;
- the monitoring of the quality of care provided;
- the review of client needs (DOH/DSS 1989, p. 211).

The concept of 'case management', as Simon Biggs has pointed out, has been imported from the United States, where it was used to improve caring by pooling resources and linking these to assessed need, thereby developing a holistic approach, defining objectives clearly. Biggs sees this as progression in the United States, but in the United Kingdom context the method is 'more a means of achieving a non-provider role for state services that would wither away, leaving the field free for entrepreneurial endeavour' (Biggs 1990, p. 3).

The Community Care Bill

The National Health Service and Community Care Bill (1989) followed from the White Paper and has begun the first phase of its implementation. The government has announced, at the time of writing (May 1991), that full implementation is to be delayed until 1993, because of financial restrictions. As noted above, the legislation changes the role of the social worker as well as that of the local authority. Since the latter's focus is now to become the purchase of care, the social worker's responsibilities must now concentrate on assessment and case management.

From policy to practice

An early evaluation of a Community Care Programme in Practice suggests that the stress levels created for community practitioners may be high. The key worker role, for example, has an intensity 'which brings its own stresses and strains' (PSSRU 1990). Further confusion arises from the relationship between the roles of the key worker and the care (or case) manager. Can the roles be identical? Some would argue that the White Paper has moved the key worker focus away from the client, since its emphasis was not cost-effective management. Barry Meteyard, author of *The Community Care Key Worker's Manual*, argues, that as a consequence, the care manager could not possibly be anyone outside of the managing authority (the Social Services Department), 'that it must be someone away from the grassroots of care, someone distinct from those closest to the client' (in Redding 1991).

Local authority interpretations of case management indicate a fair amount of variation. The magazine *Community Care* has compared Devon Estover SSD with Cheshire. This comparison illustrated considerable differences between the two areas in terms of client groups covered; multi-agency finance and the involvement of care managers in service provision (although in Devon there seems to have been no final decision reached) (Neate 1991). Care management for the highly dependent elderly has recently been introduced in Kent, where care management models themselves are well-developed. The emphasis here is on 'tailor-made packages' of care, designed with the involvement of the client, and the early evidence suggests that the 'Kent Model' has been received favourably and is working well (Community Care 1990).

Such findings indicate both a well-known truism in policy matters; namely, that there is always variation in practice, at local level, and that some locally developed systems can become models of 'good practice'. Nevertheless, this should not blind us to the ways in which such new and positive practices are inextricably linked to a concern with financial management and cost effectiveness. As Simon Biggs notes, there is a continuing emphasis on delegated budgets, the monitoring and evaluation of performance and the like (Biggs 1990, p. 29). This emphasis points to the government's belief in marketing and choice at 'the point of sale' and stresses a 'managerialist' approach to the problems of limited resources and identifies a shift from a professional 'provider culture' to the culture of 'enabling' and 'brokering'.

The concept of choice

It is worth taking a close look at the concept of *choice*. This concept is acknowledged in a good deal of the talk about, and the literature on, community care. As Eric Midwinter has recently argued, *real* choice for the consumer-citizen (a notion which embraces the carer as well as the cared-for) hinges on *informed* choice, that is, the capacity to choose between a range of alternatives, based on sound knowledge and education (Midwinter 1991). The distinction the consumer-citizen, as distinct from the consumer, is not merely semantic. Midwinter is arguing here for the centrality of the person(s) who receive services, in terms of their democratic participation, as citizens with rights, in the process of determining the nature of that service. This insight shifts the whole axis of the community care debate towards the actual *consequences* of care, and forces us to ask questions like has there been a real, positive outcome for the consumer-citizen? Midwinter sees this as a new and significant departure from the (by now) rather sterile debate between the over-bureaucratised tendencies of traditional forms of collective provision and the emphasis on public expenditure cuts and 'choice' from the political right.

To make such participation a reality may entail a shift in power away from local authorities towards service users. As Linda Ward suggests, service users should be involved in their own assessments and care packages. The impetus for this involvement, however, has been stifled by the government's failure to implement sections 1–3 of the Disabled Persons Act 1986, which would have facilitated advocacy and consultation for disabled persons (Ward 1991).

This points out the complex interdependence between policy areas, which often has a bearing on effective implementation. Ward argues that users need to be involved in inspection units, service audits and other mechanisms concerned with quality of service, if the rhetoric of community care is to become a reality.

The relationship between community care and income maintenance policies is of similar significance. Saul Becker has forcefully put the case that the level and availability of Social Security benefits will be crucial determinants of the effectiveness of community care. Since so much of the work of SSD's is created by inadequate benefits, the implications for community care are that many of the most vulnerable user groups, such as discharged psychiatric patients, will be unable to participate in 'normal' and customary activities (Becker 1990). There are echoes here of Peter Townsend's conception of what it means to be poor – the lack of opportunity to partake fully in the life of the community (Townsend 1979).

The carers

The other consumer-citizens, equally in need of full democratic participation, are carers. There are approximately six million carers in Britain. This six million represents a figure much higher than those numbers caring for children under 5 years of age at home, and about half are over retirement age. As Jill Pitkeathly points out, many carers are, themselves, in their eighties and even nineties. This group often tends to be ignored by policy-makers and certainly has little electoral 'clout' (Pitkeathly 1990a). Fears have often been expressed that due to demographic and social changes, such as the impact of rising divorce and re-marriage rates restructuring the patterns of family obligations, the future supply of carers may 'run dry'. Yet even if such fears are unfounded, little heed is paid to the very real needs of such people. Jill Pitkeathly has reinforced the point about carers' need for recognition and involvement, arguing that many professionals still see carers in the role of recipient of services, rather than as knowledgeable partners (Pitkeathly 1990b). Perhaps the primary help that carers need though, is adequate cash benefits, (a) to support their caring, and (b) to compensate them for the opportunities forgone in the labour market.

The black community

The final aspect of the consumer–citizen relationship to community care to be examined in this chapter is that of black people. The initial difficulty here is how to recognise the culturally specific needs of black people through the legislation. Like the early development of mainstream voluntary groups, black voluntary groups emerged as a response to the gaps left by statutory provision (Duorado 1991). Ways of working with and within black communities, however, do not readily relate to the approaches identified in the Community Care White Paper and legislation. Approaches from the local authority to a local voluntary group to provide a contracted, specialised service, for example, run the risk of alienating the voluntary group by threatening to incorporate it into the statutory mainstream of provision. Further, as Duorado (1991) points out, the holistic approach to care, claimed for the Community Care Act, is close to the usual ways of working of many black voluntary agencies, which refuse to compartmentalise the community into the conventional statutory classifications. It remains to be seen whether and how far the formal rhetoric of the policy-makers can bridge the gap to the community-centred approaches of black people. The legislation and much of the policy literature, has been so often revealed to be gender-blind; can it overcome its tendency to race-blindness and ethnocentricity too?

Clearly, the many different minority ethnic groups in Britain are likely to have differing conceptions of community care and it will be incumbent upon those involved with service delivery to be attuned to this important cultural diversity. Tony Acland deals with these issues of race and culture more extensively in the next chapter, but here we wish simply to highlight some of the implications for implementation of community care policy.

Within the ethnic minority population (of 2,580,000) (Labour Force Survey 1989) there is a particular profile which needs to be considered in relation to community care. Men outnumber women among the black elderly, for example, due to differences in migration patterns (LGIU 1991). It has been recognised for some time that black people are over-represented in psychiatric hospital admissions (Klug and Gordon 1983) and there persists, of course, the problem of language and communication between the social services (and other agencies) and many minority groups. This problem needs to be addressed through initiatives like 'mother-tongue' social workers and demands a new approach which will have resource implications.

In terms of the proposed new 'contractual' relationship between the social services departments and voluntary bodies the Local Government Information Unit points to the dangers of the shift towards 'mixed economy of care', suggesting that the impetus towards large-scale cost-effective private companies will mean that the locally based, ethnically sensitive, voluntary bodies will be displaced, and that the former will not be orientated towards the specific needs of the minority community (LGIU 1991).

Conclusions

The issue of race highlights some of the central difficulties involved with the policy implementation of community care. It reminds us that Britain is now, clearly, a *multi-cultural, multi-ethnic* society. We are a diverse society and one which has experienced a rapid rate of change, socially, economically and culturally, in the post-war period.

The central question, it seems, is whether the ways in which community care policy has evolved, the ways in which it is spoken of, written about and discussed, the policy intentions themselves, are matched with, and are appropriate to, the reality of the social lives we now lead.

For example, will married women with child-care responsibilities, beckoned back to work by employers seeking a 'flexible' workforce, be willing to consider the role of carer when financial and material support is uncertain? Have social work departments fully addressed the possibility of racist assumptions and attitudes within social work practice? What are the implications for social work recruitment and training? Perhaps, above all, we might ask, have we cultivated a set of social values conducive to caring? Have we not permitted the values of the market and of competition to pervade our thinking at all levels? This is an important question, since, as we noted at the beginning of the chapter, 'caring' as an activity and as a thought process, relies on and is rooted in genuine altruism and concern for others. These ideas are increasingly difficult to hold to, or aspire to, when evidence, both from academic research and of our own eyes, seems to remind us of how divided our society is. David Donnison has recently written of the 'new poverty' which, by its very nature, has the effect of marginalising more groups than ever before from the mainstream activities of the society, and deepens the divisions 'between those in the core and on the margins of the labour force' (Donnison 1991).

We cannot somehow hope to implement 'care in the community', to emphasise *caring* for *people*, whilst at the same time denying people access to the experience of taking control over their own lives, by creating fulfilling work and educational opportunities for them, by ensuring that all contributions to our society and its reproduction are properly recognised and resourced, and, above all, by empowering people, through giving them access to decision-making processes, and by treating them as adult consumer-citizens. This may sound like pure wish fulfilment, and we are certainly not suggesting that 'throwing money at social services' is any kind of solution, but these issues of *values* and of realising genuine citizenship, need to be addressed if the rhetoric of community care is not to become yet another lost opportunity.

Policy analysis – a practical exercise

The acid test of any analysis is whether or not it can shed light upon a real-life situation. If the preceding analysis is able to enhance understanding of the policy process as it affects the work of the community worker, then it will have met its objective.

In order to apply the analysis the following exercise is suggested:

1. Try to obtain some literature from your local authority on its plans for care in the community. (This should be readily available from social services departments, clinics, post offices, etc.)
2. Study it carefully and try to assess its stated objectives. You might also try to 'read between the lines' of the text to discover any gaps or ambiguities in provision.
3. Compare your study of this policy literature with your own experiences and observations of actual practice:
   (a) Is there a *gap* between policy objectives and the reality you experience on a daily basis? What are the reasons for this?
   (b) Is the policy merely '*symbolic*', i.e. just rhetoric with no concrete proposals?
   (c) What are the actual *outcomes* for your clients?
   (d) Can you identify the *obstacles* in the way of the effective *implementation* of community care policy?

References

Barret, S. and Fudge, C. (eds.) (1981) *Policy and Action*. London: Methuen.

Bayley, M. (1973) *Mental Handicap and Community Care*. London: PKP.

Bayley, M. (1978) Community oriented systems of care. Berkhamstead Volunteer Centre.

Becker, S. (1990) The sting in the tail, *Community Care*, 12 April.

Biggs, S. (1990) Consumers, case management and inspection: obscuring social deprivation and need? *Critical Social Policy*, Winter.

DHSS (1971) Cmnd 4683, London: HMSO.

DHSS (1975) Cmnd 6233, London: HMSO.

DOH/DSS (1989) *Caring for People: Community Care in the Next Decade and Beyond*. London: HMSO.

Donnison, D. (1991) *Squeezed and Broken on the Brink*. THES, 19 April.

Duorado, P. (1991) Getting the message across, *Community Care*, 21 May.

Evans, N. (1990) In Savage, S. and Robins, L. (eds.) *Public Policy under Thatcher*. Macmillan.

Finch, J. (1982) *Exploring Society*. In Burgess, R. (ed.) London: British Sociological Association.

Giddens, A. (1987) *Social Theory and Modern Sociology*. Polity Press.

Goffman, E. (1961) *Asylums: Essays on the Social Situation of Mental Patients and Other Inmates*. New York: Doubleday.

Glouberman, S. (1991) The pit and the pendulum: an inside story. *The Guardian*, 16 January, p. 21.

Griffiths, R. (1988) *Community Care – Agenda for Action*. London: HMSO.

Halsey, A. H. (1990) Who cares anyway? *Analysis*. BBC Radio 4, 9 December.

Ham, C. and Hill, M. (1984) *The Policy Process in the Modern Capitalist State*. Wheatsheaf Books.

Jaehnig, W. (1979) *A Family Service for the Mentally Handicapped*. London: Fabian Society.

Jones, K. (1989) Community care: old problems and new answers. In Carter, P., Jeffs, T. and Smith, M. (eds), *Social Work and Social Year Book I 1989*. Milton Keynes: Open University Press.

King, J. (1990) A helping hand, *Community Care*, 22 February.

Klug, F. and Gordon, P. (1983) Different worlds. Runnymede Trust.

Langan, M. (1990) Community care in the 1990s: The Community Care White Paper, Caring For People, *Critical Social Policy*. Autumn.

Local Government Information Unit. The Black Community and Community Care.

Lunn, T. (1989) Will the terms be right? *Community Care* (Supplement), 30 November.

Meteyard, B. (1991) In Redding, D. The key to success, *Community Care* (Supplement), 28 March.

Midwinter, E. (1991) Community care? community life (lecture given at the University of Southampton), 7 May.

Ministry of Health (1966) *Health and Welfare*. Cmnd 3022. London: HMSO.

Neate, P. (1991) Putting it into practice, *Community Care* (Supplement), 28 March.

Open University (1984) Social polical and social welfare. Block 4, Unit 13. Milton Keynes: Open University Press.

Parker, R. (1981) Tending and social policy. In Goldberg, E. M. and Hatch, S. (eds.) *A New Look at the Personal Social Services*. London: Policy Studies.

Pitkeathley, J. (1990a) Who cares anyway? Institute analysis. BBC Radio 4, 9 December.

Pitkeathley, J. (1990b) Painful conflicts, *Community Care* ('Inside'), 22 February.

PSSRU (1990) Care in the community – lessons from a demonstration programme. No. 9, May 1990. University of Kent.

Seebohm, F. (1968) Report of the committee on local authority and allied personal social services (the Seebohm Report). Cmnd 3703. London: HMSO.

Townsend, P. (1979) *Poverty in the United Kingdom*. Penguin.

Walker, A. (1982) The meaning and social division of community care. In Walker, A. (ed.) *Community Care*. Basil Blackwell/Martin Robertson.

Ward, L. (1991) Having a say in community care, *Community Care*, 11 April.

Wolfensberger, W. (1972) The principle of normalisation in human services. Toronto: Canadian National Institute for the Mentally Retarded.

Chapter 3

Sociological issues: family, gender, community, class and race

Tony Acland

1. Introduction

The aim of this chapter is to demonstrate the contribution of sociology in developing community practitioners' understanding of their clients as members of diverse social groups. Using ideas and research drawn from a wide range of sociological enquiry, this chapter explores issues which are important for all who administer care in the home of their clients – the nature of family life, gender relations, community life, social class and ethnicity.

It is not the purpose of this chapter to cover all the sociological literature of relevance to the community practitioner. Rather, by illustrating the usefulness of sociology to community practitioners, it is hoped to encourage further reading in order to increase understanding of clients as members of complex social groups.

2. The nature of sociology and its importance to community practitioners

Sociology has been defined in a number of ways, reflecting the diverse nature of approaches and research methods used by sociologists. Indeed, any attempt to provide a single definition which claims to encapsulate the full spectrum of sociological enquiry runs the risk of concealing, rather than revealing, the special nature of the different approaches which constitute modern sociology. Perhaps, the most useful general definition, which recognises the wide range of sociological enquiry, has been provided by Anthony Giddens[1]:

> Sociology is the study of human social life, groups and societies. It is a dazzling and compelling enterprise, having as its subject matter our own behaviour as social beings. The scope of sociology is extremely wide, ranging from the analysis of passing encounters between individuals in the street up to

the investigation of global social processes (Giddens 1989, pp. 7–8).

Each of the major sociological approaches has a contribution to make for community practitioners who wish to improve their understanding of the clients whom they will encounter. In this chapter, we will draw on the functionalist, social conflict, feminist, social action and interpretist approaches in order to illustrate the usefulness of sociology to the work of the community practitioner.

The functionalist approach

This approach examines society as a functioning social system in which all the parts of the system, people and different social institutions, are interrelated to form a stable and cohesive social entity. Based on the ideas of early sociologists, such as Emile Durkheim[2], functionalists assume that social cohesion and stability are the normal state of affairs in society for two reasons:

1. in an increasingly specialised world, people depend upon each other to perform particular roles, e.g. doctor and baker. The same is true of social institutions where, for example, the courts and the custodial services are *functionally interdependent*; and
2. because powerful socialisation agencies, such as the family, organised religion, educational institutions and the mass media, function to inculcate *shared values and beliefs* which bind people together and integrate communities.

In recent years, the functionalist approach has been the subject of considerable criticism[3]. It has been accused of uncritically accepting the importance of value consensus and the maintenance of the current social order, as well as failing to adequately examine the causes of social change, unrest and deviance. Whilst recognising the potency of such criticisms, the functionalist approach is useful to the community practitioner:

- by focusing attention on the whole community as a functioning *social system*, it emphasises the importance of viewing the client as part of an *integrated* (or *disintegrated*) *community*. The professional's attention is focused upon the whole network of community positions, roles, rights and responsibilities which affect the client's health and welfare; and
- it examines the *important functions served by social institutions*, such as the family and religious organisations, for society and individuals within it.

Radical sociology: the social conflict and feminist approaches

Radical sociologists adopt a critical perspective and question the role of social institutions, such as the family or traditional gender roles. They point to the way in which many social institutions oppress their members and can generate stress and social problems. They also note that certain social class, ethnic and gender groups are disadvantaged in a number of aspects of their lives, including their experience of health and welfare.

In contrast to functionalism, the social conflict approach emphasises the fundamental *differences* which exist between social groups. Based particularly on the work of Karl Marx[4], they note the unequal nature of a society in which privileged social classes enjoy the lion's share of the available wealth, housing, health and other resources. Because of their different economic and power positions in society, different social classes are seen to possess contradictory economic interests. According to the social conflict approach, such a situation will inevitably lead to the creation of quite different attitudes and beliefs and make conflict between social classes inevitable.

Feminists also reject the functionalist image of a stable, cohesive society based on shared values and beliefs. Instead, they critically focus upon the disadvantaged position of women in society, hoping to play an active role in changing the inequalities which their research reveals. According to Maureen Cain[5], being a feminist means '. . . interacting with other women who are working towards a transformative understanding of women's condition'. As Caroline Ramazanoglu[6] explained, taking a feminist standpoint necessitates a rejection of the positivist research principles of detached analysis and disinterest in policy recommendations. Feminists, she argued, must be politically engaged in order to produce knowledge of social life which is not otherwise discoverable.

These radical approaches are useful to the community practitioner:

- Their emphasis on *social differences*, particularly in terms of economic interests, warns the professional to avoid simple generalisations concerning clients' needs. Clients from different socio-economic backgrounds may perceive their health and welfare needs in a quite different manner from that expected by the community practitioner.
- The focus on *social inequality* encourages the health professional to identify the links between health experience and gender, race and the socio-economic background of the client.

Social action and interpretist approaches

Advocates of these approaches reject the attempt by other sociologists to study social structures and broad patterns of social behaviour. Influenced by writers such as Max Weber[7] and Husserl[8], attention is centred upon the *individual* as a social actor.

In advancing the social action approach, Weber argued that social behaviour could only be understood by examining the way in which individuals *interpet* their social circumstances. Interpretist sociologists, such as Aaron Cicourel[9], are less concerned with explaining behaviour, viewing sociology as an attempt to *describe how individuals make sense of their social world.* They advocate the adoption of a participative and intuitive approach to the study of the *social meanings* which individuals create in particular social settings.

This type of sociology is important to the professional working in the community:

- It encourages the health professional to 'take nothing for granted' and to investigate how individual clients build a commonsense understanding of their medical condition, treatment and the roles of community practitioners whom they encounter.

In this chapter, sociological research influenced by all of the above approaches will be used to illustrate the way in which sociology can assist the community practitioner in meeting the special challenges of working outside of a hospital setting.

Exercise

Different sociologists view the social world in contrasting ways. How many different perceptions of clients have you noticed amongst your colleagues?

3. The sociology of the family

No other branch of sociology demonstrates the contrasts between sociological approaches more than the field of family studies. However, before examining these competing approaches it is important to identify the way in which families and households have changed in recent years.

Demographic trends and family relationships

Data available from the Central Statistical Office[10] reveal demographic trends which are certain to affect family relationships:

- By 1987, one-person households constituted 25% of all households, compared to 12.5% in 1961.
- One-parent families have risen from 7% of all families in 1971 to 14% by 1987.
- By 1988, Britain had the second highest divorce rate in Europe – 12.3% of existing marriages.
- In less than 10 years, cohabiting by couples between the ages of 18 and 49 increased from 3.3% (1981) to 7.7% (1988).
- Births outside marriage have risen from 12% in 1981 to 27% in 1989.

The above trends, coupled with the continued ageing of the population, raise serious questions concerning the ability of the familial ties to provide effective care for the young, elderly and chronically sick in British society. This suggests that there will be a growing need for the services of community practitioners.

Changes in the family structure

Sociological analyses of the changing structure of the family have done little to allay the fears of those who predict the increasing inability of the family to care for its dependent members. In their comparative analysis of the diverse family patterns in fourteen European countries, Katja Boh and associates[11] noted that whilst the family remained an important institution, families throughout Europe had to constantly adapt to the growing conflict between home and work. Family members, they predicted, would come under increasing pressure as they attempted to cope with the competing pressures between their domestic and working roles. Similarly, in Britain, the Rapaports[12] noted the growth of 'dual career families' in which both adult partners pursued full-time careers in a way which challenged the traditional division of labour between the sexes.

Some sociologists anticipate a shift in family roles in which men and women share the burden of domestic and child care responsibilities to meet the pressures of modern society, without necessarily placing greater demands upon the community practitioner. For example, Young and Willmott[13] predicted the growth of the symmetrical family where family members of different ages and both sexes enjoy a greater measure of equality and share decision-making and roles in a manner unknown in the past.

However, such predictions have not gone unchallenged. For example, Stephen Edgell[14] found little evidence that young middle class couples shared domestic and child care roles, despite Young and Willmott's suggestion that structural change would begin within the affluent middle class and be diffused to other social groups. Whilst further research will be needed to resolve this particular issue, this sociological debate is useful, because it centres attention on the nature of power, equality and role differentiation within the home – issues which no community practitioner can afford to ignore when negotiating an effective health care programme.

Functionalism and the study of the family

Functionalist sociology has paid special attention to the study of the family because it believes this social institution to have a central role in creating and maintaining social cohesion and stability. Murdock[15], the American functionalist, pointed to the universal existence of the family in order to demonstrate the vital *functions* which the institution served for society and the individual. This view is shared by the influential British sociologist Ronald Fletcher[16]. Fletcher argued that the importance of the functions served by the family in contemporary society has not diminished. Indeed, he claimed that these functions have increased in importance. Not only have legal reforms (in areas of public health, education and economic provision) increased the burden of responsibility on parents; but modern communications have enabled family members to preserve links across geographic boundaries. Fletcher argued that in the late 1980s the family continues to:

- regulate sexual behaviour;
- provide for protection, sustenance and care of children, the disabled, the sick and the elderly;
- provide education for members in the youngest and most crucial years, thereby maintaining community customs, traditions and morality.

If functionalist analysis is correct, the burden on community practitioners will not significantly increase. Indeed, community practitioners can treat families as a significant resource to draw upon in the performance of their professional duties.

Another important contribution of functionalism is to encourage the analysis of the family as a fully functioning *social system*. The family is seen as a set of interrelated positions and roles, each of which serves vital functions for the whole. The functionalist approach is holistic, arguing, for example, that we can only understand the role of an individual family member by focusing on the whole family and identifying the nature of the links between each part of the system[17].

Using such a systems approach, Bernstein[18] made a useful distinction between positional families and person-orientated families. He described the former as closed systems in which family members attempted to reduce contacts with the outside world to a minimum (with obvious implications for the challenges to the professional working in the community). Such families, he argued, aim to maintain stable and ordered patterns of authority, with family roles clearly differentiated on gender and age lines. In contrast, person-orientated families maintain a loose (and, therefore, more accommodating for community practitioners) relationship with the outside world. Such families emphasise the importance of the individual and advocate less rigid role differentiation. In a similar manner, Kantor and Lehr[19] developed an elaborate classifications of family systems. Amongst the many family systems identified, they highlighted the existence of 'Random Family Systems' which maintain dispersed, irregular and fluctuating relationships. Such families which, by definition, are so unpredictable, present special challenges to the community practitioner.

Radical approaches to the study of the family

Marxists and feminists have criticised the functionalists for failing to focus upon the *conflicts* and *problems* generated within families. For example, the Marxist writers Coontz and Henderson[20] point to the dominance of males in the family and argue that the cause of this can be traced to the difference between the roles of men and women in the production of goods. Jan Pahl[21] found that, far from protecting individuals, the family is often a source of violence and oppression for women. Summing up the view of many, Laing[22] argued that the family is a political arena where individuals 'play games' and struggle for power and dominance, with inevitable harmful psychological consequences for all family members. From this perspective, the family is more likely to generate clients for community practitioners, than provide an effective support service.

The interpretist approach to the study of the family

The interpretist tradition has produced one of the most interesting and potentially useful approaches – the study of *family life*. Pioneered by Jon Bernardes[23], this perspective challenges the conventional approach to the study of the family as a social institution. Through analysis of the 1981 census data, Bernardes claims to have exploded the myth of the existence of a stable, normal family structure. For example, Bernardes noted that only 9.8% of families conformed to the mythological model of a nuclear family (one-family households containing first-time married couples with dependent children, with the husband in full-time work and the wife not working). Bernardes urges the abandonment of this fruitless attempt to study family structure. Instead, he advocates a new approach which focuses on the complexities of family life, involving the analyses of the different meanings which individuals attach to different aspects of such life.

The importance of the study of family life to the community practitioner lies in its emphasis upon the *social meanings* which individuals attach to crises in their family lives. Bernardes pleas for research of this kind on marital strife, divorce, family violence and child abuse, arguing that this '. . . needs to be directed at increasing pleasure and reducing pain in family life'[24]. One interesting example of this new family life sociology is the analysis of adultery in modern society by Annette Lawson[25]. Although we should exercise caution in generalising from her work (because Lawson used a self-selected sample of adulterous men and women), her work does suggest that attitudes towards love, marriage and sexual fidelity are changing radically. She claims that a convergence of attitudes between the sexes is occurring in Britain. Men are joining women in the pursuit of romantic love, whilst many women are adopting the promiscuous patterns of sexual behaviour which used to be more frequently associated with men.

Exercise

Interview a colleague with at least 15 years of experience of working in the community. Ask your colleague to identify the main ways in which families and family support have changed.

4. Gender, social change and caring relationships

Perhaps the most rigorous analysis of gender roles in the home and employment have been produced by feminist writers. Their work has important implications for the nature of caring relationships in the home.

Gender inequality in the home

Michelle Barratt[26] has emphasised the way in which patriarchy (male domination of power positions in society) and gender socialisation have maintained the 'traditional' role of daughters and wives as the main providers of care and domestic labour at home. Such a situation, she argued, has prevented women from securing equality at home and in the workplace. Similarly, Anne Oakley[27] cited considerable evidence to demonstrate that the sexual division of labour in the family is not 'natural' as the functionalists claim; but that gender roles are culturally generated. She noted that girls learn (often at their mother's knee) to adopt sex-appropriate behaviour at home and work. Oakley argued that the oppression of women in the home would eventually be eradicated by a women's movement dedicated to the abolition of the family, marriage and the housewife role[28]. If Oakley is correct in this prediction, this will seriously challenge the state's current reliance on women as the main providers of care for the elderly, young and infirm.

Women as victims of stress

Feminists argue that women experience considerable stress which can be attributed to the pressure to conform to gender roles. Hannah Gavron[29] found that women of middle and working class backgrounds, who cared for their children on a full-time basis, experienced a *sense of isolation* and *imprisonment* in the home.

Such stress can lead to low levels of physical and mental health. For example, in an attempt to explain the rising incidence of alcoholism amongst women, the Camberwell Council on Alcoholism[30] blamed the new burdens on women's lives. They argued that young women feel caught between contradictory social pressures. The 'modern woman' is expected to be a supportive wife and mother, as well as to achieve a successful career in the work place. Faced with such conflict, some women turn to alcohol or drugs as a crutch for their psychological difficulties.

Gender inequality in employment

When assessing the stresses on modern women, attention should be given to the way in which British women continue to be disadvantaged in employment. For example:

- The gap in average income between men and women has recently increased, with women earning only 71.2% of men's pay in 1988, compared to 75.5% in 1977[31].

- Women may have been disproportionately affected by unemployment during the current recession in a manner not recognised by the official statistics[32].
- Women continue to be under-represented in the powerful, high status posts in the UK when compared with other Western societies[33], with female employment concentrated in the unskilled manual and low status servicing roles. Even in the social services, a caring profession which has traditionally been associated with women, men have increasingly enjoyed a disproportionate share of the senior posts available[34].

Perhaps the widespread economic exploitation of women is best illustrated by a brief examination of home work, in which pay levels are traditionally extremely low. Typically, home workers are self-employed and enjoy little protection under the law, in terms of working conditions and security of employment. Shelley Pennington and Belinda Westover[35] noted that married women engaged in home work in order to '. . . earn money and not contradict the assumptions about their domestic role'. For this reason, many women from ethnic minority groups in Britain are home workers. Sheila Allen's[36] research documented the long hours worked by such women, noting that young children were often involved. Home work is a particularly important issue for community practitioners, because it is frequently conducted in unhealthy and unsafe conditions, with inevitable consequences for the health and well-being of women and children.

The feminisation of the workforce: implications for caring roles

Despite the continuation of gender inequality in employment, an important social trend in recent years has been the increasing feminisation of the workforce. In 1987 women accounted for 45% of the workforce, compared to 42% in 1979[37]. Martin and Roberts'[38] important study of nearly 6,000 women of working age found that female attitudes to work were changing, with the majority of younger women attributing greater importance on employment. Indeed, according to the authors, the experience of marriage actually increased women's desire for work.

We should be cautious, however, before assuming that the feminisation of the workforce threatens the traditionally caring role of women. For example, for all age groups in Martin and Roberts' sample, the majority of the women (60%) thought that mothers with pre-school children should not work. In fact, only 27% of mothers with pre-school children in the sample worked, though most intended to resume paid employment when all the children had started school. Of course, children are not the only dependants affected by the growing trend of female employment, and the consequences of changing female attitudes and behaviour towards paid employment needs further research to determine future effects for the care of the elderly, handicapped and the chronically ill.

Daughters and the care of the elderly

An important area of research for community workers is the analysis of the daughter–parent relationship. In a society in which 95% of the elderly still live in their own homes, daughters continue to be their main carers[39]. However, analysis of demographic trends shows that the ratio of these potential carers (women aged 50–59) compared to the 75-plus age group has declined. In 1901 there were 2.77 potential carers for every person over 75 years of age; but in 1986 there was less than one potential carer (0.86) for every person over 75 years of age[40]. These statistics graphically illustrate the increased burden of care facing daughters in modern Britain.

Perhaps of even greater concern to those interested in the care of the elderly is evidence from recent research focusing on the *content* and *quality* of the relationships between elderly dependants and their daughters. For example, O'Connor[41] conducted a study of 60 married women (aged between 20 and 42 years) in order to critically examine the common assumption that strong emotional bonds and supportive relationships exist between working class women and their mothers in London. In contrast to the findings of Young and Willmott[42] 30 years earlier, visiting and social interaction between mothers and their married daughters was found to be infrequent. Although some degree of practical support did take place, the study showed that 'disappointment, resentment and guilt' often characterised such relationships. From the daughter's position, a bundle of negative attitudes and consequent stress formed a central aspect of the mother–daughter relationship. An important implication of this study is that there is a growing need for the daughter-carer to receive professional support, particularly as more women find themselves to be the sole carer in the family network.

Other studies have examined the effects of the rising divorce and remarriage rate on women's traditional caring role. For example, Finch and Mason[43] examined the impact of divorce and remarriage on care for the elderly in Manchester. Noting that, after natural daughters, daughters-in-law were the main carers of the elderly, the authors attempted to establish the level of care after divorce and the establishment of new relationships. Their research demonstrated that sustained caring relationships were rare, only occurring if there was a special history of emotional attachment between the daughter and parent-in-law before the divorce and if the divorcees had been able to sustain a good relationship. Such research serves to emphasise the way in which growing divorce and remarriage rates may radically influence the traditional family caring relationships in our society, placing increasing demands on the community practitioner.

Exercise

Ask your male and female colleagues who have partners in paid employment: (a) when both partners work, should they share domestic and caring tasks? (b) What proportion of domestic/caring tasks is actually shared?

5. Community, neighbourhood and social networks

The term 'community' has been used in many different ways by sociologists. Indeed, Hillery[44] was able to identify 94 different definitions. However, as Azarya[45] has noted, there has been a tendency for recent sociologists to use the concept to refer to a *collectivity* in which a group shares:

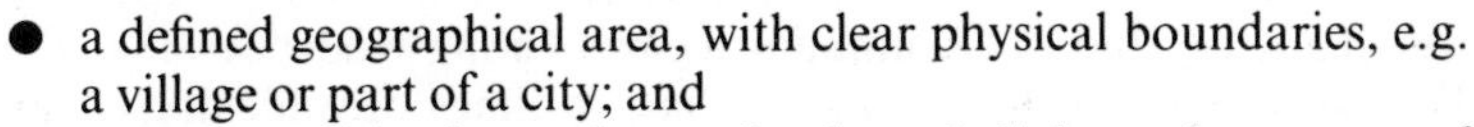

- a defined geographical area, with clear physical boundaries, e.g. a village or part of a city; and
- a common identity and set of values, beliefs, and patterns of behaviour.

The neighbourhood effect

Evidence exists to show that the locality in which people live can influence a wide range of social attitudes and behaviour, even amongst those from different socio-economic backgrounds. For example, Dickens'[46] research showed that a 'neighbourhood effect' existed in political voting preferences in certain localities, with working class and middle class people adopting common political beliefs. Dickens argued that, whatever their social class, people living in the same locality are likely to develop common ideas and beliefs, because they share similar material positions.

Dickens' analysis is useful, particularly as it explains how neighbourhoods respond to common threats, such as those caused by major road developments or the decision to close maternity hospitals. Some radical sociologists, such as Castells[47], have gone further than Dickens, predicting that urban neighbourhoods will form the basis of major urban political movements. However, it is important to recognise Gans'[48] cautionary note that urban neighbourhoods are often composed of people from a wide range of social backgrounds. Based upon his research on American suburbs, Gans suggested that lifestyles were largely influenced by social class or stages in the family cycle, rather than by locality.

Social networks

The concept of social network is not new; but is of considerable importance for those wishing to understand the nature of informal social relationships. In anthropology the concept can be found in the early work of Radcliffe-Brown[49]. In sociology it was central to Elizabeth Bott's[50] pioneering analysis of conjugal roles. More recently, Martin Bulmer[51] argued that the term 'social network' is useful for '. . . enabling one to talk about a wider set of informal relationships than just the family or the extended kin group'. He noted that the term had been broadened to include the analysis of the interconnections between friends, neighbours and work associates. Bulmer sees social network analysis as lying at the heart of the revival of community studies in the 1980s.

According to Bulmer, social network analysis is particularly useful in the study of community care. Citing evidence from the Barclay Report[52], Bulmer noted that, in times of difficulty, when family support is unavailable, people tend to turn to local informal networks rather than use the formal social services. In order to serve the local community, the Barclay Report advocated the need for all community practitioners to:

- develop detailed knowledge of their local networks; and
- establish a partnership between social networks and the formal caring agencies.

Similarly, Collins and Pancoast[53] encouraged American community workers to identify and use 'natural neighbours' or 'central figures', individuals who have sufficient energy and are strategically placed in the 'natural networks' to offer informal care and support.

The analysis of social networks is of particular importance to the health professional working in the community. This is because a number of studies have demonstrated that social networks can affect patterns of health and pathology. For example:

- Brown and Harris[54] found that *supportive networks helped to reduce levels of depressive illness*; and

- Berkman and Syme[55] demonstrated that *a relationship existed between the nature of social ties and mortality rates.*

However, the way in which social networks influence health patterns remains to be identified. As Bulmer[56] observed:

> though the association between support and outcome is established for many pathological conditions, the *precise causal factors* operating are obscure [emphasis added].

Exercise

Discuss with an experienced community nurse the extent to which she/he is able to work with neighbours to provide effective care for clients.

6. Social class differences, inequalities and health experience

When John Major succeeded Margaret Thatcher as Prime Minister in December 1990 he made it clear that he wished to create a *classless society*. Whilst this statement left many puzzled concerning John Major's personal definition of social class, the publicity which this statement received revived interest in two important issues concerning the nature of social class in Britain:

- the extent to which social class *inequalities* have been eradicated in all aspects of life, including health experiences;
- the way in which attitudes (including attitudes towards health care), beliefs and behaviour *differ* between social classes.

Before we can examine the nature of class inequality and differences in Britain we need to establish what is meant by social class. Sociological perspectives differ in the way in which they approach this issue. Perhaps, the simplest definition of social class was provided by Karl Marx, founder of the Social Conflict perspective. As Giddens[57] noted, Karl Marx viewed social class in fundamentally economic terms:

> a class is a group of people who stand in a common relationship to the *means of production* – the means by which they gain their livelihood.

For Marx, there were two major economic classes: the bourgeoisie or capitalists, who owned the means of production, and the proletariat, who possessed only their capacity to work (labour power). A central feature of the class relationship for Marx was the exploitation of the proletariat. The capitalist system, based on competition and the endless pursuit of profits, requires the bourgeoisie to *exploit* the proletariat, who, in turn, are forced to sell their labour in order to subsist. As a consequence of such reasoning, the social conflict perspective adopts a controversial position concerning the preservation of social inequality in modern society. They argue that:

- The modern capitalist economy demands *the maintenance of social inequality* in all aspects of life, because the economic system is based upon the exploitation of the working classes.
- Despite the attempts of religious bodies and the media to prevent it, the conflicting economic interests of the social classes will inevitably generate *contrasting social attitudes and political beliefs*, with the proletariat dedicated to overthrowing the capitalist system.

Ironically, the functionalist tradition also considers the persistence of social class inequalities as serving the function of preserving the current social structure. However, unlike the Marxists, they do not view this situation with alarm and do not expect such inequalities to lead to conflict and disorder. Davis and Moore[58], for example, argued that the differential allocation of economic resources in a complex social stratification system encourages and rewards people according to their skills and the relative importance of their occupation for the efficient functioning of society.

The social action tradition, founded by Max Weber, has led to a broadening of the concept of social class. Weber[59] noted that groups differ according to their position within a number of market situations, of which the employment market was only one. From this perspective, an adequate understanding of social class must examine differential access to power, status, leisure and economic opportunities. This approach emphasises the differences between social classes in terms of lifestyles, attitudes and behaviour in a manner which makes it the closest sociological approach to that adopted by the Registrar General in the classification of official statistics according to the supposed social standing of occupational groups in society[60]. Although officially abandoned in 1987, because of criticisms regarding its reliability and validity[61], the Registrar General's classification remains the main basis for research on social class inequality and difference in lifestyle.

Before examining the nature of class inequality and difference, it is important to note that there has been a growth in the size of the non-manual workforce and a decline in manual jobs during the 1980s. Between 1989 and 1990 the number of non-manual jobs increased by 3.2%, whilst manual jobs declined by 2.0% in the same year[62]. At this time, 51.4% of the male workforce were in manual occupations, with 48.6% in non-manual jobs[63].

Between 1945 and 1979 there was a steady growth in the standard of living of all classes in Britain, with inequalities of income and wealth being slowly reduced in size. However, since 1979, inequalities of income and wealth have widened. According to the government publication, *Social Trends*[64]:

- In 1987 the wealthiest 20% of households received 39.1% of total net income in Britain, compared to 34.3% in 1979.
- The wealthiest 10% of the population owned 53% of the country's total marketable wealth in 1988, 3% more than 10 years earlier.

Social class inequality in health experience: the evidence

One issue has dominated the debate concerning the nature of social inequality in post-war Britain: social class differences in health experience. The 1982 *Black Report*[65] confirmed the suspicions that social class inequalities of health experience persisted despite the introduction of the Welfare State in 1948. Among the many statistics cited in the report, Sir Douglas Black and his team noted that:

- the self-reported rate of long-standing illness for unskilled manual females was two and a half times that of the rate for their professional counterparts;
- males and females of the unskilled manual class had two and a half times more chance of dying before retirement than those in the professional classes;
- despite an overall decline in mortality rates, differences in the infant mortality rate between the social classes had actually widened during some periods of the post-war era;
- inequalities existed in the utilisation of health services. Whether because of under-provision of services or their attitudes to health care, working class groups used the preventative service far less frequently than the middle classes.

As Hilary Graham[66] has noted, a degree of caution should be exercised when interpreting statistical analyses which combine social class and health experience. However, the findings of the *Black Report* demonstrate the nature of the major challenges facing all who work in the health service, particularly at times of severe budgetary constraints. In particular, the evidence of the differential use of preventative health services serves to emphasise the importance of the *teaching role* of community practitioners in the area of prevention as well as general health care.

A number of studies have confirmed the findings of the *Black Report* and demonstrated that class differences in health experience persist throughout Europe, particularly amongst the vulnerable groups in society[67]. In one such study, *The Health Divide*[68], Margaret Whitehead noted that class inequalities were compounded by the existence of considerable regional discrepancies in the provision of services for the elderly and handicapped. For example:

- the ratio of home-helps to people over 75 years of age varied from 7:1000 in Cleveland to 70:1000 in Devon.

Explaining social class differences in health experience

Despite the abundance of evidence demonstrating the existence of inequality in health experience, more research is needed to establish the causes of health inequality. The *Black Report* discussed four competing explanations:

- The idea, advanced by the government in 1980, which dismisses inequality findings as mere *artifacts*, pieces of statistical accident or trickery with little basis in reality.
- The *natural or social selection* argument[69] whereby occupational class is seen as the result of differential health experiences, as filtered through different generations, i.e. the healthy become upwardly mobile and the unhealthy become downwardly mobile.
- The *materialist or structuralist* explanation[70] which, pointing to inequalities of wealth and income, blames the deprived material environment of the unskilled manual classes for their high mortality and morbidity rates.
- The *cultural/behavioural* explanation[71] emphasises the health consequences of different attitudes and behaviour of the social classes. For example, differences in dietary practices and smoking[72] are explained by examining contrasts in education or custom.

Whatever the relative merits of the four explanations, the artifact and natural selection approaches permit little opportunity for intervention by the health authorities. On the other hand, the explanations offered by the materialist and cultural approaches provide a sounder basis for the development of effective strategies for the removal of inequalities in health experience, particularly through improved education, housing and welfare provisions. For the individual community worker, these analyses serve to emphasise the importance of the intricate relationships between health experience and their clients' material and cultural circumstances.

Exercise

Consider your own clients and identify contrasting attitudes between individuals from different social classes. In particular, have you noticed different attitudes in the way in which they view your role as a community practitioner?

7. Race, ethnic differences and inequalities

Immigration and race relations

Immigration has long been a feature of British society. However, as Ellis Cashmore[73] observed, until 1948 there were relatively small numbers of non-white residents in Britain (about 10,000, many living in the Liverpool area). From June 1948 until the early 1970s, when legislation restricted immigration, there was a steady influx of immigrants, at first from the Caribbean and later Asians from India, Pakistan, Bangladesh and African States. According to the 1981 census, the number of Asian immigrants alone had risen to 750,000, plus dependants. By the end of the 1980s approximately 6% of the British population was non-white.

Social conflict writers such as the Marxists Miles[74] and Castles and Kosack[75] observed that increased immigration was encouraged by government and firms in the 1950s and 1960s to provide large quantities of cheap labour for the expanding capitalist economy. They noted that discrimination and exploitation of ethnic minorities by employers was widespread. In sharp contrast to the analysis of functionalist writers, such as Patterson[76], Marxists predicted that racial hostility from white workers would increase, particularly as economic crises generated competition for jobs.

The urban riots of the 1980s, particularly in Bristol, Brixton, Toxteth and Handsworth, led many to examine the relationship between ethnic minorities and government agents, notably the police, education and welfare services. Benyon and Solomos[77] observed that the main cause of the riots was *a profound sense of injustice* felt by inner city residents. Rioters, not all of whom were non-white, believed themselves to be discriminated against, exploited and rejected by the establishment in Britain. Even the offical report by Lord Scarman[78] recognised that many non-whites experienced such a deep sense of alienation and rejection by society that they lashed out at the police and distrusted all representatives of the establishment.

The above analysis demonstrates the challenges facing community practitioners in the establishment of client relationships, based on trust and mutual respect, in Britain's inner city areas.

Racial discrimination and inequality: the evidence

The evidence concerning the pervasiveness of racial discrimination and inequality is extensive. In the first major study of racial discrimination in Britain, Daniel[79] noted that:

> There is racial discrimination [in Britain] varying in extent from massive to the substantial.

Despite repeated attempts by governments to outlaw racial discrimination through the Race Relations Acts of 1965, 1968 and 1976, research, such as Smith's[80], continued to demonstrate the existence of widespread discrimination, particularly in employment opportunities. A major report in 1985, *Faith in the City*[81], noted the appalling rate of unemployment and sense of hopelessness and alienation amongst the young black population in British cities, laying much of the blame for this situation on the failings of the government and government agencies.

According to a PSI Report[82], even non-whites lucky enough to be economically active experience discrimination, particularly in terms of promotion at work and in the running of their own businesses. Phizacklea and Miles[83] observed that, despite their proud record of supporting the British trade union movement, Afro-Caribbean and Asian workers had received little practical union support in the fight against racial discrimination.

As Ahmed, Cheetham and Small[84] have emphasised, it is important for all professionals working in the community to understand that, '. . . racism bears so hard on the lives of black people and . . . is at the root of so many problems'. The authors noted that *minorities even experience racism from professional people*, which, in turn, affects their behaviour towards all community practitioners whom they meet. Ahmed noted that stereotyped beliefs about minority families have even influenced the behaviour of trained social workers, and pointed to incidents where social workers have prematurely intervened to remove children from black households because of the mistaken view that the parents were overstrict and unable to adapt to a changing environment. The authors observed that, given the considerable power of social workers and other professionals, it was vital for community practitioners to attempt to obtain a detailed understanding of their client's cultures.

Ethnic minorities: the diversity of life-styles

Studies of particular communities demonstrate not only the diversity of life, but also the ability of groups to adapt to new environments, in a manner which defeats simple ethnic stereotypes. In Acland's[85] analysis of a small Hindu community in a Midlands town, different Asian individuals displayed a diverse range of behaviour towards other groups in the town. Dependent upon their different status ambitions within the Asian community, some attempted to maximise their social relations with white groups (appearing to integrate), whilst others sought to segregate themselves totally from all other ethnic groups. Shaw's[86] study in Oxford demonstrated the ingenuity of Pakistani families in adapting their Islamic way of life to the restrictions of their small English houses. In order to observe the ideals of Purdah, which requires the segregation of females from males for part of family life, these Islamic families created a system whereby, for example, females shared the front room with the males, only vacating it on the arrival of a male visitor.

These studies demonstrate the importance of a sound knowledge of clients' customs, together with a positive attitude towards ethnic differences. It is particularly important for community practitioners to:

- acquaint themselves with the medicinal and dietary practices of different ethnic groups in their client population[87];
- avoid making simplistic assumptions about the ways of life of minority groups. Generalisations, for example, about 'the Asian way of life' can damage effective relationships with clients; and
- avoid viewing the cultural traditions of minority groups as social weaknesses which must be overcome. On the contrary, the characteristics of a particular group may be useful to both the professional and the client in the negotiation of an effective health care programme.

Exercise

Consider your own experience of health care (in the community or hospital setting) and identify examples where current professional practice could be modified to meet the social needs of ethnic minority groups.

8. Conclusion: putting sociology to the test

The main objective of this chapter has been to illustrate the importance of sociology as a means of improving community practitioners' understanding of their clients as members of diverse social groups and economic circumstances. Using ideas and research drawn from different sociological perspectives, the chapter has explored the nature of family life, gender relations, community life, class and ethnicity.

However, the proof of the pudding is in the eating. In order to determine the usefulness of sociological analysis to a specific client situation, the following exercise may be attempted:

Exercise: conducting a social audit of a client group

Aim
To identify the social characteristics and diverse nature of a specific client group.

Procedure
Using the sociological ideas discussed in this paper, analyse your client group according to the following characteristics:

Family characteristics

e.g. Identify the proportion of clients with carers. Determine the relationship of carers to the client, i.e. proportion of daughters, daughters-in-law, other carers.

Gender characteristics

e.g. Determine the range of attitudes towards gender roles, with special reference to providing care for the elderly.

Community characteristics

e.g. Establish the extent to which clients consider themselves to be members of a tight-knit community or social network, with a pattern of mutual rights and responsibilities.

Social class characteristics

e.g. Identify the proportion of clients in each of the Registrar General's socio-economic groups. Compare the attitudes of each group towards preventative health care.

Race and ethnic characteristics

e.g. Identify the proportion of clients in distinctive ethnic groups. Consider similarities and differences in their approach towards health care.

Notes

1. Giddens, A. (1989) *Sociology*. Oxford: Polity Press.
2. Durkheim, E. (1947) *The Division of Labour in Society*. New York: The Free Press.
3. For a brief and balanced summary of criticisms of Functionalism, see Michael Haralambos (1990) *Sociology: Themes and Perspective* (3rd edn) pp. 778–781. Oxford: Polity Press.
4. For a useful selection of Marx's original work, see Bottomore, T. B. and Rubel, M. (eds) (1966) *Karl Marx: Selected Writings in Sociology and Social Philosophy*. Harmondsworth: Penguin.
5. Cain, M. (1986) Realism, feminism, methodology and law, *The International Journal of the Sociology of Law*, **14,** 225–267.
6. Ramazanoglu, C. (1989) Improving on sociology: problems of taking a feminist standpoint, *Sociology*, **23,** (3), 422–442.
7. For a useful selection of Weber's work, see Gerth, H. and Mills, C. (1948) *From Max Weber*. London: Routledge and Kegan Paul.
8. Husserl, E. (1931) *Ideas*. London: Allen and Unwin.
9. Cicourel, A. (1968) *The Social Organization of Juvenile Justice*. London: Heinemann.
10. *Social Trends*, 21, 1991, Central Statistical Office, HMSO.
11. Boh, K. *et al.* (eds) (1989) *Changing Patterns of European Family Life*. London: Routledge and Kegan Paul.
12. See, for example, Rapaport, R. G. and Rapaport, R. (1982) *Families in Britain*. London: Routledge and Kegan Paul.
13. Young, M. and Willmott, P. (1975) *The Symmetrical Family*. Harmondsworth: Penguin.
14. Edgell, S. (1980) *Middle Class Couples*. London: Allen and Unwin.
15. Murdock, G. P. (1949) *Social Structure*. New York: Macmillan.
16. Fletcher, R. (1988) *The Shaking of the Foundations: Family and Society*. London: Routledge and Kegan Paul.
17. See Morgan (1985) *The Family, Politics and Social Theory*. London: Routledge and Kegan Paul, for an excellent summary of the systems approach in the study of the family.

18. Bernstein, B. (1971) *Class, Codes and Control*, vol. 1. London: Routledge and Kegan Paul.
19. Kantor, D. and Lehr, W. (1973) *Inside the Family*. San Francisco: Jossey Bass Inc.
20. Coontz, S. and Henderson, P. (eds) (1986) *Women's Work. Men's Property*. London: Verso.
21. Pahl, J. (1978) *A Refuge for Battered Women*. London: HMSO.
22. Laing, R. D. *et al.* (1976) *The Politics of the Family*. Harmondsworth: Penguin.
23. Bernardes, J. (1990) The family in question, *Social Studies Review*, September 1990.
24. Bernardes, J. (1990) op cit., p. 33.
25. Lawson, A. (1988) *Adultery*. Oxford: Basil Blackwell.
26. Barrett, M. and McIntosh, M. (1982) *The Anti-social Family*. London: Verso.
27. Oakley, A. (1982) *Subject Women*. London: Fontana.
28. Oakley, A. (1974) *Housewife*. London: Allen Lane.
29. Gavron, H. (1966) *The Captive Wife*. London: Routledge and Kegan Paul.
30. Camberwell Council on Alcoholism (1980) *Women and Alcohol*, London: Tavistock.
31. *New Earnings Survey (1970–1988)*, part A, tables 10 and 11.
32. Lewis, J. and Bowlby, S. (1989) Women's inequality. In Herbert, D. T. and Smith, D. M. (eds), *Social Problems and the City*. Oxford: Oxford University Press.
33. See, for example, Davidson, M. J. and Cooper, C. L. (eds) (1984) *Working Women. An International Survey*. New York: Wiley.
34. Skinner, J. and Robinson, C. (1988) Who cares? Women at work in social services. In Coyle, A. and Skinner, J. *Women and Work*. London: Macmillan Education Ltd.
35. Pennington, S. and Westover, B. (1989) *A Hidden Workforce*. London: Macmillan.
36. Allen, S. and Wolkowitz, C. (1987) *Homeworking*. London: Macmillan.
37. *Department of Employment Gazette*, April 1991, vol 99, no. 4.
38. Martin, J. and Roberts, C. (1980) *Women and Employment: a Lifetime Perspective*. London: HMSO.
39. See, for example, Wenger, G. (1984) *The Supportive Network: Coping with Old Age*. London: Allen and Unwin.
40. Bulmer, M. (1987) *The Social Basis of Community Care*. London: Unwin Hyman.
41. O'Connor, P. O. (1990) The adult mother/daughter relationship: a uniquely and universal relationship? *The Sociological Review*, **38,** 293–327.
42. Young, M. and Willmott, P. (1961) *Family and Kinship in East London*. Harmondsworth: Penguin.
43. Finch, J. and Mason, J. (1990) Divorce, remarriage and family obligations, *The Sociological Review*, **38,** 219–246.
44. Hillery, G. A. Jr (1955) Definitions of community: areas of agreement, *Rural Sociology*, **20**(2), 111–123.
45. Azarya, V. (1989) *The Social Science Encyclopedia*. London: Routledge and Kegan Paul.
46. Dickens, P. (1988) *One Nation? Social Change and the Politics of Locality*. London: Pluto.
47. Castells, M. (1977) *The Urban Question*. London: Edward Arnold.
48. Gans, H. (1967) *The Levittowners*. London: Allen Lane.
49. Radcliffe-Brown, A. R. (1940) On social structure, *Journal of the Royal Anthropological Institute*, 70.
50. Bott, E. (1957) *Family and Social Network*. London: Tavistock.

51. Bulmer, M. (1987) op cit., p. 109.
52. Barclay Report (1982) *Social Workers: their Role and Tasks (Report of a working party under the chairmanship of Mr P. M. Barclay)*. London: Bedford Square Press.
53. Collins, A. H. and Pancoast, D. L. (1976) *Natural Helping Networks: a Strategy for Prevention*. Washington DC: National Association of Social Workers.
54. Brown, G. W. and Harris, T. (1978) *The Social Origins of Depression: A Study of Psychiatric Disorder in Women*. London: Tavistock.
55. Berkman, L. and Syme, L. (1979) Social networks, host resistance and mortality, *American Journal of Epidemiology*, **109,** 187–204.
56. Bulmer, M. (1987) op cit., p. 126.
57. Giddens, A. (1990) op cit.
58. Davis, K. (1967) Some principles of stratification. In Bendix, R. and Lipset, S. (eds), *Class, Status and Power* (2nd end). London: Routledge and Kegan Paul.
59. Gerth, H. and Mills, C. (1948) op cit.
60. Originally designed in 1911, the Registrar General's classification is based on an individual's *general standing in the community*. By the 1960s six main groups were used:
    A – Professionals and senior managers of large firms, e.g. lawyers, general managers.
    B – Semi-professions and middle managers, e.g. teachers, executives in the civil service.
    Ci – Skilled non-manual, e.g. clerk.
    Cii – Skilled manual, e.g. plumber, miner.
    D – Semi-skilled manual, e.g. machine operator.
    E – Unskilled manual, e.g. labourer.
61. See, for example, the excellent critical discussion of the Registrar General's classification system in Reid, I. (1977) *Social Class Differences in Britain*. Open Books.
62. 'The 1990 Labour Force Survey Preliminary Results', reported in *The Employment Gazette*, April 1991, **99** (4), 175–204.
63. 1990 Labour Force Survey, op cit.
64. *Social Trends*, 21, 1991. London: HMSO.
65. Townsend, P. and Davidson, N. (1988) *Inequalities in Health: the Black Report* (3rd edn). Harmondsworth: Penguin.
66. Graham, H. (1984) *Women, Health and the Family*. Hemel Hempstead: Harvester Press.
67. See, for example, Fox, A. (ed.) (1988) *Inequalities in Health within Europe*. London: Gower.
68. Whitehead, M. (1986) *The Health Divide*. London: Penguin.
69. For a critical discussion of this argument, see Goldberg, E. and Morrison, S. Schizophrenia and social class, *British Journal of Psychiatry* (1963), **109,** 785.
70. See, for example, McKeown, T. (1979) *The Role of Medicine*. Oxford: Basil Blackwell.
71. See, for example, Fuchs, V. (1974) *Who Shall Live? Health, Economics and Social Choice*. New York: Basic Books.
72. In 1988, 43% of males from the unskilled manual class smoked regularly, compared to 16% of males from the professional classes (*Social Trends*, 1991).
73. Cashmore, E. E. (1989) *United Kingdom? Class, Race and Gender since the War*. London: Allen and Unwin.
74. Miles, R. (1982) *Racism and Migrant Labour*. London: Routledge and Kegan Paul.
75. Castles, S. and Kosack, G. (1973) *Immigrant Workers and Class Structure in Western Europe*. Oxford: Oxford University Press.

76. Patterson, S. (1963) *Dark Strangers: A Study of West Indians in London*. Harmondsworth: Penguin.
77. Benyon, J. and Solomos, J. (1987) *The Roots of Urban Unrest*. Oxford: Pergamon Press.
78. See, for example, Scarman, L. (1982) *The Scarman Report*. Harmondsworth: Penguin.
79. Daniel, W. W. (1968) *Racial Discrimination in Britain*. Harmondsworth: Penguin, p. 209.
80. Smith, D. (1977) *Racial Disadvantage in Britain*. Harmondsworth: Penguin.
81. Church of England (1985) *Faith in the City: the Report of the Archbishop of Canterbury's Commission on Urban Priority Areas*. London: Christian Action.
82. Brown, C. (1984) *Black and White Britain: The Third PSI Report*. London: Heinemann.
83. Phizacklea, A. and Miles, R. (1987) The British trade union movement and racism. In Lee, G. and Loveridge, R. *The Manufacture of Disadvantage*. Milton Keynes: Open University Press.
84. Ahmed, S., Cheetham, J. and Small, J. (1986) *Social Work with Black Children*. London: Batsford.
85. Acland, T. (1989) Integration and segregation in an Asian community, *New Community*, **15**(4), 565–576.
86. Shaw, A. (1988) *A Pakistani Community in Britain*. Oxford: Basil Blackwell.
87. See, for example, the collection of useful articles in Cheetham, J. *et al* (eds) (1991) *Social and Community Work in a Multi-Racial Society*. London: Harper and Row.

Suggested reading

The nature of sociology

Haralambos, M. (1990) *Sociology: Themes and Perspective* (3rd edn), pp. 1–23. Unwin-Hyman.

The family and family life

Allan, G. (1985) *Family Life: Domestic Roles and the Social Organisation*. London: Blackwell.

Fletcher, R. (1988) *The Shaking of the Foundations*. London: Routledge and Kegan Paul.

Laing, R. *et al.* (1976) *The Politics of the Family*. Harmondsworth: Penguin.

Gender and inequality

Graham, H. (1984) *Women, Health and the Family*. Hemel Hempstead: Wheatsheaf.

Oakley, A. (1982) *Subject Women*. London: Fontana.

Walby, S. (ed.) (1988) *Gender Segregation at Work*. Oxford: Oxford University Press.

Community, neighbourhood and social networks

Bulmer, M. (1987) *The Social Basis of Community Care*. London: Unwin Hyman.

Dickens, P. (1988) *One Nation? Social Change and the Politics of Locality*. London: Pluto.

Wenger, G. (1984) *The Supportive Network*. London: Allen and Unwin.

Class differences, inequalities, health

Townsend, P. *et al.* (1988) *Inequalities in Health: the Black Report.* 3rd edn. Harmondsworth: Penguin.
Fox, A. (ed.) (1988) *Inequalities in Health within Europe.* London: Gower.
Cashmore, E. (1989) *United Kingdom? Class, Race and Gender since the War.* Part 1. London: Allen and Unwin.

Ethnic studies

Ahmed, S. *et al.* (1986) *Social Work with Black Children.* London: Batsford.
Cheetham, J. *et al.* (1981) *Social and Community Work in a Multi-Racial Society.* London: Harper and Row.
Shaw, A. (1988) *A Pakistani Community in Britain.* Oxford: Basil Blackwell.

Chapter 4

Legal issues

Howard Davis

Introduction – the kind of legal issues to be dealth with

In this chapter we examine some relevant issues of law. The aim is to consider a range of legal issues that can arise from the fact that a person is working in the community. Our concern is with the legal significance of happenings that are more likely to occur when a person is working, for example, in a private dwelling or in a small residential home, rather than in a hospital or similar institution.

We do not discuss the legal framework within which health and welfare services are provided. To do so would alter our focus on matters which relate specifically to working in the community. Nor are general professional matters, such as the duty to patients or questions involving contracts of employment, dealt with; these should be covered in general training and are discussed in, for example, Andrews (1991).

The law is introduced in a general way and is not examined in detail. If you read this chapter you will not become a lawyer but you will better understand some aspects of your legal position as a practitioner providing services in the community; furthermore, you will better be able to recognise situations in which it might be a good idea to get legal advice.

The chapter has three sections.

Section A deals with situations in which health practitioners may suffer harm to themselves or their property as a result of working in the community and how their rights to compensation may be affected.

Section B involves a consideration of various circumstances in which health practitioners may be liable for harming others in the course of working in the community.

Section C relates to ancillary issues involving legal matters which are not directly connected with a person's work but which might be of importance given his or her presence in the community.

Section A. Losses sustained by a community health practitioner

Introduction

Health professionals, like other workers, may be harmed in the course of their work. Usually this harm will be in the form of physical injury or illness or damage to personal property. The legal system provides a means by which such a person can obtain redress, usually financial compensation, for his or her loss. Whether a person has a right to redress depends upon the law relating to workers' health and safety. This is vast and complicated. A full general account is to be found in Smith and Wood (1989), Chapters 10 and 11; updated detail is contained in the *Encyclopedia of Health and Safety at Work*.

In this section we consider, at a general and non-technical level, those aspects of the law which are particularly relevant to community work.

1. Contract and state benefits

Where a person is injured at work it is often enough to rely on the various benefits which arise under his or her contract of employment or which are available from the government as welfare state benefits.

(a) Benefits under the contract of employment

Many community health practitioners are employees of the National Health Service and, on the basis of their employment contract, can benefit from the NHS Sick Pay Scheme and the NHS Injury Scheme. Entitlements under these schemes are the same whether the work is done in the community, in a hospital or some other place. If a health practitioner is employed by other bodies, such as GP partnerships, NHS Trusts or by charities, the terms and conditions of employment should be checked for comparability against those offered by the NHS.

(b) Welfare state benefits

A community practitioner injured through work is also entitled to a range of welfare state benefits. These may be for injury, disease, disablement etc. Benefits for such 'industrial injuries' are based on proof that the 'employed earner suffered personal injury caused . . .

by an accident arising out of and in the course of employment'. As with benefits under the contract, the availability of welfare state benefits does not depend on whether or not the work is in the community. However, the benefits are taken into account when calculating the sum payable under the contractual schemes and so will not increase the amount of money available. Detail of welfare state benefits can be found in Ogus and Barendt (1988).

2. Compensation for negligent actions

The contractual and welfare state benefits mentioned above are sufficient for many persons who are injured or made ill through work. The problem is that although these benefits mainly provide a regular income related to normal pay, they will often not be adequate to compensate for a range of other losses that may flow from serious injury or illness. For example, they will not compensate for medical and other expenses, pain and suffering, distress, loss of life expectancy or for the more expensive ways of life that may result from disablement; nor will they provide compensation for the loss of valuable property.

(a) Negligence in general

To obtain such compensation it is usually necessary for the injured person to prove that the injuries resulted from someone's negligence. Proving negligence can often be difficult. It means showing, on a balance of probabilities, that someone was at fault in the sense that her or she failed to guard against risks that a reasonable person in that position would have foreseen and taken steps to prevent. In court the injured person (the plaintiff) must show, first, that he or she was owed a duty of care by the person who injured him or her (the defendant). In respect of personal injury and damage to property, it is normally enough to show that the plaintiff was someone that the defendant should have had in mind as likely to be affected by his or her action and that harm was reasonably foreseeable. Second, the plaintiff must show that the defendant was in breach of the duty of care. This means that the defendant failed to act reasonably in all the particular circumstances. An important point to note is that the defendant need only have guarded against reasonable probabilities; failing to prevent something which is no more than a remote possibility is not negligence. Third, the plaintiff must show that his or her injuries were caused by the defendant's breach of a duty of care. For a full account of the tort of negligence see, for example, Brazier (1988).

(b) Vicarious liability

In all torts, including negligence, the person sued (the defendant) is not necessarily the person who actually caused the harm. Under the principle of vicarious liability an employer is liable for the negligence of his or her employees. This means that the person harmed (the plaintiff) is more likely to get the compensation he or she is entitled to since it can come from the employer's insurance or greater resources. Employers are liable without it being shown that they are themselves at fault; thus even if the plaintiff's loss was caused by actions which the employer had forbidden, the employer can still be liable.

(i) Course of employment
Vicarious liability only applies where the employee was acting in the course of employment; if the employee was doing something unconnected with his or her employment the employer will not be liable.

(ii) Independent contractors
Similarly, if the losses are caused by an independent contractor, not an employee, the remedy will normally be against the contractor rather than the person or organisation employing him or her even if that organisation is better placed to pay damages than the contractor. There are exceptions to this general rule; for example, if the employing organisation is engaged in dangerous work they cannot usually escape liability for injuring others simply because the injuries were caused by the negligence of their independent contractor.

(iii) Indemnification
The employer has a right to seek indemnification from the employee; this is not usually done unless the employee is covered by their own insurance as, for example, physiotherapists are covered by the indemnity policy of the Chartered Society of Physiotherapy.

(iv) NHS employees
Where injuries are caused to patients and others by the negligence of medical staff the liability of the NHS is clearly established; it is based either on vicarious liability or on breach of a direct legal duty to patients.

On the basis of these general points about negligence we shall now consider some particular issues that may affect community health practitioners.

3. Employers' liability

Workers who are injured or who catch a disease as a result of their work will normally look first for compensation from their employer. Employers have various health and safety duties towards their employees and ought either to have sufficient funds or to carry insurance to meet successful claims by their employees. The fact that a person is employed by a publicly funded body will not normally affect the issue. A district health authority, for example, is in the same general legal position as a private employer regarding the health and safety of its employees.

Two general points about the legal position of employers and employees should be noted. Under their contract of employment, employees need only obey orders which are reasonable. A community practitioner, therefore, is unlikely to have a contractual duty to attend at a place known to be hazardous or where criminal attacks are foreseeable. In reinforcement of this, the courts have held that health authorities can withdraw services if their duty to a patient is outweighed by their duty to protect their staff from criminal attacks or lesser forms of abuse (Wyatt 1977).

Employers can be liable to pay compensation to their employees on two main grounds. The first is that the employer is in breach of a statutory duty; the second is that the employer is liable in negligence – directly, for being in breach of the common law duty of care, or vicariously liable as where when one employee injures another. There are, however, a number of difficulties regarding workers in the community whose job is performed in places which are not under the supervision of their employer.

(a) Breach of statutory duty – regulations

Under the Health and Safety at Work Act 1974 and other legislation, legally enforceable regulations are produced governing health and safety in many areas of work. An employer who allows a breach of these regulations may be liable to compensate an employee who is injured as a result. There are, however, no regulations relating specifically to community health practitioners, employment in domestic premises or residential homes.

(b) Employers' common law duty of care

A more fruitful source of compensation is to show that the employer is in breach of the common law duty of care owed to employees. This is a duty involving negligence and so the duty on the employer is only to take reasonable and proportionate care to avoid foreseeable risks. An employer may be liable if he or she subjects his or her employees to any risk which he or she can reasonably foresee 'and which he can guard against by any measure, the convenience and expense of which are not entirely disproportionate to the risk involved' (Harris 1953). In particular the duty relates to the provision of competent fellow employees, the provision of safe equipment and providing a safe system of work.

(c) Employers' duty regarding working in premises not under their control

(i) A duty of care is owed
The duty to take reasonable care still applies even though an employee is sent to work in premises that are not under the employer's control. The courts have accepted, for example, that a home help's employer owed a duty of care when she was injured cleaning a window in domestic premises to which she had been sent in the course of her general duties (McCloskey 1983). This duty includes taking care to avoid reasonably foreseeable dangers in the means of access as well as in the premises themselves.

(ii) The amount of care may be less
However, the courts have accepted that the amount of care the employer must show is likely to be less in respect of premises they do not control. In order to fulfil their duty, employers need only show they have taken reasonable care and the courts accept that, in respect of premises they do not control, there may not be much that employers can reasonably be expected to do.

(iii) No duty to make preliminary visits
There is, for example, no general duty to make preliminary visits and inspect premises to which employees are sent to work (Wilson 1958).

(iv) Reporting dangers
Reasonable care by an employer includes the keeping of a Hazard Book in which dangers are reported. Such a record should include the reporting of incidents of violence or the presence of dangerous dogs – matters discussed later in this chapter. Where dangers have been reported, the courts will be more willing to find that consequential harm was reasonably foreseeable. Failure by the employer to take appropriate action – such as informing the occupier of the danger or preventing their employer from attending – would be the

basis of a successful claim for damages (Smith 1959). It is important that even minor faults, such as uneven doorsteps or loose carpets, be recorded since they can be the cause of serious injury.

(v) Employees' duties

The courts accept that, to a considerable extent, employers are entitled to rely upon the good sense and reasonable skill of their employees – the more skilled and experienced the less the employer will have to do in order to discharge their duty. However, in some decisions, employers have been found in breach of their duty through not reminding employees of likely dangers and not providing them with the means to work safely to prevent foreseeable dangers materialising (General Cleaning Contractors Ltd 1953).

(d) Other remedies – general duties under the Health and Safety at Work Act

(i) General duties

Although we are looking at ways in which an injured community health practitioner can obtain compensation, it is convenient here to say a little about the general duties under the Health and Safety at Work Act 1974. This Act provides the framework for much of the health and safety regulatory law and practice. Its provisions include the imposition of general duties on employers, employees and others to ensure the health and safety of people at work.

(ii) Breach of general duty does not provide grounds for compensation

Breach of one of these duties cannot, however, provide an additional avenue for compensation. The Act provides that breach of a duty does not give a right to sue for damages; in any case, the general duties do not provide for a standard of care that is significantly greater than the reasonableness standard of negligence.

(iii) Breach of general duty is grounds for enforcement

Breach of these general duties can be the basis for intervention by health and safety inspectors who have various powers to require changes or to stop unsafe practices and even, usually as a last resort, to prosecute in the criminal courts.

(iv) Limited application of general duties to community work

Compared with a person who works at their employer's premises, a community practitioner may be at a disadvantage, particularly when working in private homes. Under the Act, an employer has a general duty to ensure as far as possible the health and safety at work of all his or her employees. This includes a duty to ensure the safety of 'places of work'. However, the duty applies only in so far as the places are within the employer's control – so community practitioners are not usually protected by this provision.

What about the owners of the places in the community where the health professional works? The Act places a duty on persons who control premises to ensure as far as possible the health and safety of all people who work in those premises. Thus those who control, for example, a residential home for children or elderly persons will owe a duty to someone, such as a health professional, coming to work there. The duty is owed even though the nurse, physiotherapist, health visitor or whoever is not employed by the controllers of the home. However, the Act expressly says that this duty is not imposed on the controllers of 'domestic premises' – so a person working in a private home cannot benefit.

(iv) Employees' duty of care

It should be noted, however, that the Act does impose a duty on employees as to their own health and safety and that of their fellow employees.

4. Occupiers' liability

In the previous section I have indicated why, because the community health practitioner is working away from premises controlled by his or her employer, compensation under the law relating to the health and safety of employees may be difficult to obtain. An alternative is to seek compensation from the 'occupier' of the premises in which the worker's loss (injury or damage to property) occurred. The occupier may be liable where the injury or damage is caused by a defect in the premises – unsafe electric sockets, slippery floors etc.

(a) Occupiers' Liability Act 1957

The Occupiers' Liability Act 1957 gives statutory force to the common law position and places the occupier of premises under a legal duty to take reasonable care to ensure that a visitor is reasonably safe in using the premises – so long as the visitor is using them for the purpose for which he or she is invited or permitted to be there.

(i) The 'occupier'
The 'occupier' is the person or organisation who, themselves or through their agents or employees, has the immediate right to control and supervise the premises. The term normally includes owner occupiers, tenants of rented accommodation, and the controllers of residential homes such as local authorities, charities or private concerns. A landlord is likely to be the occupier of common areas, stairs, lifts, halls etc. in blocks of flats. A duty to visitors is also owed under the Act by the occupier or persons having control over 'structures' – and these include accommodation such as caravans (though not the sites) and houseboats.

(ii) Damage to property
An action under the Occupiers' Liability Act 1957 extends to damage to property, including property that the visitor does not own but which he or she is entitled to bring with them on to the occupier's land – this includes employer's equipment taken into homes.

(b) The usefulness of the Act

There are a few general points about the Occupiers' Liability Act 1957 which may present obstacles to a community practitioner seeking compensation.

(i) Ability of the occupier to pay compensation
Occupiers' liability may not be of much assistance regarding work done in private dwellings. Many tenants or owner occupiers will be too poor to be worth suing – unless they are insured. Some policies for insuring the contents of houses include cover for occupiers' liability. Where a community practitioner is injured in a residential home, the occupier (a local authority, charity or private concern) is likely to have funds or insurance to cover a claim for liability.

(ii) Need to prove fault
Under the Act it is still necessary for the injured person to prove fault. It must be shown that the occupier failed to take what in all the circumstances was reasonable care.

(iii) Skilled workers are expected to guard against the risks of their calling
Under the Act, skilled workers are expected to appreciate and guard against any special risks ordinarily incident to their calling. The extent to which someone who regularly works in other people's

homes should, as a matter of professional expertise, be aware of dangers on the premises and take steps to protect themselves is unclear. For example, an occupier might not be liable to a physiotherapist who was injured as a result of plugging a machine into a defective electric socket where there was enough evidence of the defect to put a reasonably skilled operator of the machine on guard.

(iv) Dangers caused by an independent contractor

If the danger on the premises was caused by the occupier's independent contractor (a building firm, for instance) then liability usually lies with the contractor rather than the occupier. The occupier is only liable if he or she had not acted reasonably in entrusting the work to the contractor or had not taken necessary steps to satisfy themselves that the work was properly done and that the contractor was competent.

5. Animals

(a) Strict liability under the Animals Act 1971

Particular problems for community practitioners can be caused by the animals belonging to the persons they visit. The person responsible for an animal can be liable in various ways for the damage and nuisance it causes. Where a domestic animal, such as a dog, bites and injures someone, its owner could be liable in negligence. This, of course, requires evidence of lack of care which may not be the case or which may be difficult to prove. The law, therefore, provides that the 'keeper' of a domestic animal may, by virtue of the Animals Act 1971, be 'strictly' liable for injuries caused. Strict liability means that the injured person does not have to prove fault; the keeper is liable because his or her animal has caused an injury not because he or she is at fault. The 'keeper' is the owner of the animal or the person with possession. Where the animal belongs to a person under 16 years the 'keeper' is the head of the household.

For there to be strict liability:

- there must be an injury caused which is of a foreseeable kind given the animal concerned (a bite from a dog, for example);
- the animal must belong to a species which does not normally cause injury unless at certain times, like a bitch in litter or breeds of dog such as bull mastiffs which attack in defence of their territory;
- the dangerous characteristic of the particular animal must have been known to the keeper.

If these three elements are present, the keeper is liable.

There are a few defences available to the keeper. The most relevant is that the loss occurred because of the plaintiff's own fault or that the plaintiff voluntarily accepted the risk. However, a health worker who is under a duty to treat a patient and who does so despite knowing that there is a dangerous dog around, is unlikely to have 'voluntarily' assumed the risk.

(b) Other measures

The Dangerous Dogs Act 1871 gives magistrates powers in respect of a dog which is dangerous and not kept under proper control. Magistrates can order the destruction of such a dog or require the owner to take specific measures such as muzzling. For these powers to be exercised it is not necessary to show that the dog has injured any person.

Other provisions relate to dogs in public places. The Dangerous Dogs Act 1991 creates an offence of permitting a dog to be dangerously out of control in a public place or any place where the dog is not permitted to be. The same Act requires dogs of specified breeds bred for fighting to be muzzled and on a lead when in public places – including in the common parts of blocks of flats. The owners of the dogs must obtain third party insurance. At the time of writing, only pit bull terriers and Japanese tosas are restricted. The restrictions cannot be made to apply to dogs such as rottweilers and cross breeds which are not bred for fighting, even though they are as likely as any to make attacks.

6. Compensation for criminal injuries

Health professionals who work in the community may be more liable to suffer criminal attacks than those who work in hospitals. They may, for example, suffer violence in people's homes or on the street. The point of criminal law is to deter crime and punish offenders. A prosecution for a crime is brought by the Crown rather than by the victim. Nevertheless, within the criminal justice system there are procedures through which the victim can obtain compensation.

(a) Compensation from the criminal

One possibility is to seek compensation from the convicted criminal. Under the Powers of Criminal Courts Act 1973 the courts have the power to order convicted criminals to pay compensation to their victims. The compensation can cover personal injury or other loss or damage and extends to some losses caused by road traffic offences.

There are drawbacks with this procedure. It may not, for example, have been possible to prosecute and convict the criminal; criminals are often too poor and in no position to pay compensation (the means of the criminal are taken into account by the court when deciding whether to order compensation and, if so, how much to award), and, finally, the levels of compensation are not high.

(b) Compensation from public funds – the Criminal Injuries Compensation Board

A second possibility is to seek an award from public funds. Such awards are granted by the Criminal Injuries Compensation Board (CICB) which was reorganised in 1988 and whose powers can be found in s. 108–117 of the Criminal Justice Act 1988.

(i) Criminal injuries

The Board can authorise compensation in respect of 'personal injury directly attributable to a crime of violence' – these are criminal acts usually, though not necessarily, involving violence to the person. The money can be paid even if no person has been prosecuted or convicted for the offence.

(ii) Calculation of the award – the lower limit

The amount payable is based on the amount that a civil court would order to be paid as damages in respect of the same injury. However, there is a lower limit to the compensation that can be paid by the Board. In February 1990 this minimum sum payable was £750. Furthermore, the sum is calculated by taking the figure for common law damages and subtracting any social security payments which fall due. This means that injuries requiring no more than minor treatment or which have not led to more than 3 to 4 weeks absence from work are likely to fall outside the scheme.

(iii) Motor injuries excluded

Compensation is not payable for injuries caused by traffic offences (unless the victim is deliberately run down). Here the remedy is against the other driver's insurance or through the Motor Insurer's Bureau if the driver is uninsured.

(iv) Crime must be reported to the police
It is a requirement of the scheme that the victim should, unless incapable, have reported the crime to the police at the earliest possible opportunity. Merely reporting to his or her employer is not sufficient. A late report made merely to obtain compensation may lead to the rejection of an application. Applicants must also be prepared to cooperate with the police. Applications to the Board must be made as soon as possible after the incident.

(c) Civil liability of the criminal

Criminal actions will usually also be civil wrongs and the victim may sue the criminal for damages in the civil courts. The action is often going to be in the tort of trespass. Trespass relates to personal injuries and damage to property, but can include damages for the consequences of being frightened by the prospect of an immediate attack. The damages should be similar to an award from the CICB; furthermore the victim, in civil law, has the problem of finding and proving against a defendant who is worth suing. For relatively minor attacks damages are not available if the defendant has been prosecuted in a Magistrates Court – and this rule applies whether the defendant was convicted or acquitted.

(d) Employers' liability

Finally, a health practitioner could consider a civil action for damages against his or her employer under the general principles of employers' liability outlined earlier in this chapter. Employers will, however, only be liable if they have failed to take reasonable care by, for example, sending their employee to a person's home or through a street where a criminal attack was reasonably foreseeable. The courts, for example, have generally refused remedies to employees who are attacked when collecting wages or taking money to the bank where there is evidence of the employer taking some care.

As said earlier in the chapter, it is unlikely to be a breach of a health practitioner's contract of employment to refuse to attend at a place where criminal violence is foreseeable, nor, it seems, is the health authority under a duty to send an employee to such a place.

Advice from the Health and Safety Executive is that a detailed record of all incidents should be kept which can provide a factual basis for deciding appropriate policies.

Exercises on Section A

1. As a community health practitioner you attend patients at a rest home. You plug your equipment into a normal looking wall socket and are badly burned by an electric shock. Due to the severity of your injury you are off work for 10 months.

(a) On what basis, if at all, will you continue to receive all or part of your normal salary?
(b) On what basis, and against whom, might you be able to obtain compensation for your pain and suffering?
(c) What are the legal reponsibilities of your employer, the Health Authority, in respect of your safety in such places?

2. You enter Mr A's house. You are about to begin treatment on his 14-year-old son when you are attacked and badly bitten by Rambo, the son's pet labrador. Rambo is known to be aggressive when strangers approach the boy. Otherwise Rambo is well behaved, well treated and kept under control.

(a) Though there is no evidence of lack of care by the son or Mr A, on what legal basis might you still be able to obtain compensation for your pain and suffering?
(b) You report the attack to your employer. What action should be taken?

3. Your patient, Mrs B, lives in an area with a high rate of street crime. On the way to visit her you are attacked, injured and robbed by a group of youths. You recognise one of them as Mrs B's son.

(a) In what ways and from whom might you be able to obtain compensation for your losses?
(b) How will your ability to obtain compensation be affected if you decide not to involve the police because of the likely effect on Mrs B if her son is arrested?
(c) You report the action to your employer. What action should be taken; can you lawfully refuse an explicit instruction to continue treatment of Mrs B in her house; can the Health Authority lawfully refuse to continue to offer such treatment to Mrs B?

Points to consider:

1(a) Sick pay or injury scheme under the health worker's

contract of employment; alternatively, welfare state benefits under the National Insurance scheme.

1(b) Negligence. Need to prove the existence and breach of a duty of care and resulting loss. Occupiers' Liability Act – duty of care owed by the controllers of the rest home to lawful visitors – but has there been a breach of that duty?

1(c) Employer's common law duty of care in respect of the health and safety of their employees when at work. How extensive is that duty when the employee is working away from the employer's premises? Employer's general duties under the Health and Safety at Work Act 1974 – though these do not affect compensation.

2(a) 'Strict liability' and the Animals Act 1971; distinguish from negligence. Relevance of other remedies against dangerous dogs.

2(b) Reporting dangers to an employer; employer's liability for foreseeable risks.

3(a) Compensation from the criminal in the course of a criminal case; compensation from public funds; compensation from the criminal in a civil action.

3(b) Criminal Injuries Compensation Board – need to inform the police.

3(c) Hazard book; contractual right of employees to refuse unreasonable orders; health authority may balance the duty to provide care with the well-being of its staff.

Section B. Liability of a community health practitioner to others

A community health practitioner may find him- or herself liable for causing loss to others. In this section we are concerned with situations in which liability arises in circumstances likely to come about from work in the community, rather than in a hospital or similar institution. Issues such as medical negligence or consent to treatment are not covered here, since there is little of legal significance that arises particularly from community work. Such issues are briefly discussed in Andrews (1991) and in full detail in Powers and Harris (1990) and Jackson and Powell (1987, especially Chapter 6).

1. Vicarious liability – course of employment

Liability is most likely to be based on a civil wrong ('tort') or, in private practice, on a breach of contract. Where liability is in tort, the employer (the District Health Authority, for example) will be 'vicariously liable' – on the same principles as discussed in Section A2(b), above. The employer is only liable if the employee is acting in the course of his or her employment. There are a number of issues involving course of employment which relate to work in the community.

(a) Travelling

One such issue involves liability for injuries caused when travelling between different homes. Such journeys will be within the course of employment. However, journeys during the working day but which are wholly unconnected with the job are likely to be thought of as a personal 'frolic' and outside the scope of employment.

(b) Non-professional tasks

Another problem that may arise for the community practitioner is in respect of non-professional tasks which may be done for patients – bringing them a cup of tea, for example, or giving a patient or relative a lift to the shops. Such activities, if done negligently and causing injury, might not be within the course of employment – hence leaving the community practitioner themself, or their insurance company, liable.

2. Entering people's homes

(a) Trespass

Most community practitioners do not have statutory powers to enter people's homes. There are some exceptions which apply to various agencies, including the police and local authority social services departments, who have responsibilities for the health, safety and welfare of children, the mentally impaired and the elderly. Even these agencies usually only have the power to enter on the basis of a court order. Some of these matters are further discussed in section C, later.

A community health practitioner must normally have the consent of the people in possession, usually the occupier, to go on to premises. Consent to enter is given or refused by the occupier (the manager of a home, tenant, owner occupier etc.) and is not the same thing as consent to treatment which is given by the patient, or parent if the patient is a young child. If a community practitioner is asked to leave then he or she should do so; consent can be later withdrawn and to remain, like entering without permission, is a 'trespass'. Though there would be little likelihood of legal action, one consequence is that reasonable force can be used to eject a trespasser. So if a community practitioner was injured as an unintended consequence of being bundled out, he or she might find that being a trespasser made any claim for damages difficult to uphold.

(b) Preventing dangers to others

A person is not a trespasser if that person enters premises because of 'necessity' – to prevent a greater harm than the trespass creates. To perform a rescue or protect someone from immediate injury would count.

3. Damage to property

A community health practitioner may find themself liable to the patient or occupier for damaging their personal property. Usually such claims will be covered by the occupier's own contents insurance. The insurance company may, especially in relation to valuable property, require their client to bring an action against the community practitioner to minimise the sum they have to pay out. There is no liability for blameless actions – switching on a kettle which burns out due to a defect which a reasonable person would not suspect, for example. Liability is based on carelessness or intention; but, even so, liability will be found in respect of many so-called accidents.

Any action against the community practitioner will be in tort (Trespass to Goods or Negligence) and, so long as the damage was caused in the course of employment, the employer will be vicariously liable.

4. Employers' property

(a) Accidental damage

There may be increased dangers of loss or damage to employers' property which is transported about and taken into people's homes. A community practitioner, like any employee, has a duty of reasonable care and skill in respect of his or her employer's property. This is based upon a term, expressed or implied, in the employment contract. The duty is to avoid risk to property which a prudent person would foresee. Particular care should be taken in respect of any drugs or medicines that are carried, since their loss may involve dangers to the public. Similarly, special care must be taken in respect of the care of medical records, since these involve the duty of confidentiality. The question of records is discussed further in section B5.

(b) Unauthorised use of employers' property

It should be noted that the deliberate misuse of employers' property is likely to be unlawful. For example, using, without consent, NHS equipment for a private contract. It will be unlawful even if such a restriction is not expressed in the contract of employment, since the courts imply a term of faithful service, breach of which can lead to dismissal and would be of considerable weight in any adjudication of the 'fairness' of that dismissal.

(c) Gifts

Any gifts received in the course of employment become the property of the employer.

5. Records and confidentiality

Medical records, at least the paper they are written on, are the property of the NHS (Family Practitioner Committee for GP's notes, the District Health Authority for Hospital Records). The same principles of reasonable care apply to such records as to other property belonging to an employer. Regarding records, though, there is a further duty to maintain confidentiality.

(a) Duty of confidentiality is owed to the patient

The duty of confidentiality is clearly established. Community practitioners should note that the duty is owed to the person giving the information – usually the patient alone. Disclosure to spouses, cohabitees, family, friends etc. without the patient's consent is a breach of the duty. In respect of child patients, consent to disclose to a parent, for example, will need to be obtained if the child is mature enough to consent to his or her own treatment.

(b) Exceptions

There are a number of exceptions to the duty of confidentiality, such as where disclosure is required for litigation or where there is an overriding public interest or, perhaps, as in the context of AIDS, where the health of a sexual partner is at stake – such disclosures would not be for a community health practitioner by him- or herself to make.

(c) Legal consequences of unauthorised disclosure

(i) Action for breach of confidence
If an unauthorised disclosure is made the patient may seek damages to compensate for resulting losses or an injunction to restrain further disclosures. It is not always necessary to show that the disclosure would be or has been damaging; and in respect of medical information obtained in confidence, the courts recognise a very strong public interest in maintaining confidentiality. However, a court action is only likely in respect of serious disclosures where, for example, a third party such as the press or a competing business intends to make use of the information disclosed; and, in any case, the injunction may be against that third party.

(ii) Complaint to employer or professional association
A more likely course for patients is a complaint to the community practitioner's employer who could take action, including dismissal, on the basis of a breach of an implied or expressed term of the employment contract. Alternatively or additionally, a patient might complain to the appropriate professional body, the Chartered Institute of Physiotherapy for example, who could take action against a health practitioner on the basis of a breach of their professional code of ethics.

(d) Careless disclosure

A negligent or careless disclosure – leaving records in an unlocked car from where they are stolen, for example – may be sufficient for an action for breach of confidence against the community health practitioner; though most of the cases in this area involve deliberate disclosures. However, if the patient suffers resulting loss then they may be able to sue in Negligence. More probably, as with deliberate disclosures, the community practitioner is at risk from complaints to their employer or professional body who can take action for breach of contract or to enforce the code of ethics.

(e) Disclosure to patients

(i) Manual records written prior to 1 November 1991

Disclosure to the patient of the content of medical records written before 1 November 1991 is, under English law, a matter for the professional judgement of medical practitioners. Patients do not have a right to know the details of their case and community health practitioners should take care before disclosing matters which do not directly involve their own practice. The consent of the referring GP or hospital doctors should be obtained. The courts can order the disclosure of medical records in order to facilitate legal proceedings such as actions for negligence against health authorities; even here they may only permit disclosure to legal or medical advisers. Other attempts to force disclosure against resistance from doctors or health authorities may fail, with the courts upholding a public interest in protecting professional judgement of a patient's best interests.

(ii) Computer records and manual records written after 1 November 1991

Where health records are computerised they come within the scope of the Data Protection Act 1984. Patients have 'subject access rights' which include a right to be informed that personal data are being kept about them, a right to a copy of those data and a right to make corrections. The Access to Health Records Act 1990 gives patients broadly similar access rights in respect of manual health records compiled after 1 November 1991 – though child patients are excluded.

It is not clear how big a change these two Acts have introduced since patients' rights of access to both manual and computerised medical records are subject to important exceptions. In particular access rights do not apply where disclosure would be likely to cause serious harm to the physical or mental health of the person, or where disclosure would lead, directly or indirectly, to the identification of another person, other than a health professional, who has not consented to the disclosure – e.g. a person who gave information in confidence. However, even in those circumstances there is a duty to disclose whatever information can be supplied which does not have the stipulated effects.

Exercises on Section B

1(a). As a community practitioner, you are giving treatment to Mr C, a wealthy patient. You are in a hurry and, not hearing his request to the contrary, you place some equipment on to a valuable table, damaging it seriously.

(b) You attend to Miss D, a disabled patient. Having finished treatment, she asks you to make her a cup of tea – a thing you do not usually do. Due to your hurry, you spill the tea over her and she is badly scalded.

(c) You are driving to a patient's house. You cross a red light and injure Mr E, a motorcyclist.

Discuss whether Mr C, Miss D or Mr E have grounds for compensation and, if so, who may they be able to obtain the compensation from?

2. You are treating Mrs F, an adult patient. She asks to see her medical records, currently in your possession, and which you know to contain some rather insulting remarks about her.

(a) Does Mrs F have any right to see her records? How, if at all, does the position change in respect of records compiled after 1 November 1991?
(b) What would your answer to the request be if your patient was a reasonably intelligent child of 14 years?
(c) What would your answer be if Mrs F's husband, without her knowledge, asked to see her records?

3. You attend at the house of Mrs G. Her husband, who thinks she would be better served by a faith healer, refuses to let you in. You know that Mrs G wants and needs your treatment. You decide to avoid Mr G and enter through the back door. Mr G discovers your presence and strongly and firmly pushes you out of the house. As he does so you slip on the doorstep and are injured.

(a) Do community practitioners have a right to enter premises?
(b) What problems might arise in an action for damages against Mr G in respect of your injuries?

Points to consider:

1(a) Trespass to goods; negligence.

1(b) and (c) Negligence; employers' vicarious liability – whether work in course and scope of employment.

2(a) Professional decision whether to disclose. Access to Medical Records Act 1990 and its exceptions.

2(b) Position of children under Access to Medical Records Act 1990.

2(c) Duty of confidentiality owed to patient.

3(a) and (b) The tort of trespass – who gives permission to enter? Reasonable force to remove a trespasser.

Section C. Ancillary issues

In the course of community work a health professional may come across situations where others are acting illegally or where the intervention of others, police or welfare agencies, for example, may be appropriate. In this section some relevant aspects of the law are outlined.

1. The illegal actions by others

A community health practitioner may find themself present when a crime has been committed (a fight, for example) or become aware that a crime has been committed (e.g. that there is stolen property or illegal substances in a home he or she is visiting).

(a) No duty to prevent an offence

Normally a person is not under any legal duty to do anything in these circumstances. It is, for example, not aiding and abetting an offence merely to be present at the scene of a crime and to do nothing to prevent it. Aiding and abetting an offence requires some degree of active encouragement.

(b) No duty to report – exceptions

There is no general legal duty to report crimes to the police. However, it is an offence to impede the apprehension or prosecution of a person who has committed an 'arrestable offence'; likewise it is an offence to agree not to disclose information about an 'arrestable offence' in exchange for money or other gain. 'Arrestable offences' include but are not confined to the more serious offences.

There is an exception to the general principle against requiring disclosure which applies to information about acts of terrorism connected with the affairs of Northern Ireland. Failure to disclose such information to the police is an offence under the Prevention of Terrorism Act 1989.

Finally, there is no general legal requirement to answer police questions and a refusal is not in itself an obstruction of the police in the exercise of their duty.

2. Children suffering significant harm

Community practitioners may, in the course of their duties, come across a child who seems to be suffering or is likely to suffer 'significant harm'. They should consider whether to report the matter. The relevant agencies are the local authority's Social Services Department or the NSPCC (the police, also, may act in an emergency). Any report will be treated in confidence. These agencies have various statutory powers. In particular, they may seek judicial authority for a range of actions including short term emergency measures, supervision of the child at home or the permanent removal of the child from its parents. Any action taken must have the welfare of the child as its paramount concern.

If such a report is made, it must be followed up by the local authority, which is under a statutory duty to make inquiries in order to determine whether or not some action to protect the child is made. The powers of the agencies relate to children suffering or likely to suffer 'significant harm'. This means that, to a significant degree, the child is being ill-treated (including sexually abused) or its physical or mental health, or its physical, intellectual, emotional, social or behavioural development is being impaired. The law is complex, it has been recently reformed and is now mainly contained in the Children Act 1989.

3. Vulnerable people

In the course of their work community practitioners may come across people, adults or children, who, through age or handicap, are in need of help. A range of services are available. These include both residential accommodation and a considerable range of support services such as practical assistance in the home, help with laundry facilities or the provision of special equipment. Most of these services are provided through local authority social services departments. This is a large and complicated area of law which is outside the scope of this chapter.

In some circumstances a vulnerable person's living conditions will be such that it may be in their best interests to be removed, even against their will, to better accommodation where they can be looked after. There is a power to do this under s. 47 of the National Assistance Act 1948. The power is exercised by the medical officer of health or community physician of the district council who may apply to magistrates for an order. Magistrates must be satisfied that the person involved is suffering from a 'grave chronic disease' or is 'aged, infirm or physically incapacitated' and is 'living in insanitary conditions'; in all cases magistrates must also be satisfied that the 'person is unable to devote to themselves, and is not receiving from other persons, proper care and attention'. Even then the person can only be removed if it is in their interests or if removal will prevent injury to someone else's health, or prevent a serious nuisance to others. The power is a strong one and the person concerned may find it difficult to resist – though they do have a right of appeal. It is, apparently, a power that is rarely used.

4. Mentally disordered

Community practitioners may come across persons (for example, patients, their relatives, their neighbours or people in the street) whose behaviour indicates a mental disorder and a need for treatment. The majority of such people choose or are persuaded to accept hospital treatment voluntarily. There are, however, legal powers to compel persons into hospital. Such compulsory admissions may be for assessment, emergency assessment or for treatment. These powers are exercised by an Approved Social Worker or the person's nearest relative and must be supported by two or sometimes one doctor. The relevant law is complex and contained in the Mental Health Act 1983.

Where a mentally disordered person is in a public place and behaving in a way which is harmful to him- or herself or others, it may be wise to call the police. The police have, in the first place, general common law powers to prevent breaches of the peace by, for example, moving a person on or by making an arrest. In respect of mentally disordered people in public places they have a statutory power to detain in a place of safety for up to 72 hours. The person must appear to be mentally disordered, be in a public place and be in need of care and control; detention must be in their interests or to protect others. A public place has been broadly defined as any place to which the public have access, and this includes the common areas of blocks of flats such as landings. Where a mentally disordered person is in private premises and is not receiving proper care, it is open to any person to apply to magistrates for a warrant for a forced removal, by police, to a place of safety. Usually, but not necessarily, such applications will be made by relatives or approved social workers.

Exercises on Section C

1. In a rest home you notice a storeroom which contains a large number of videos marked with the own brand of a well known departmental store. You know the store has been recently burgled and you suspect the videos are stolen. The owner of the rest home realises your suspicions and offers you £1,000 to keep quiet.

(a) What legal duties, if any, do you have to the police and the public in the circumstances?
(b) Would your answer be different if you saw what you believed to be bomb-making equipment and the owner of the rest home had an obvious interest in the affairs of Northern Ireland?

2. (i) A child patient makes allegations to you that his parents are abusing him;

(ii) a patient of yours lives by herself and over the months has noticeably retreated into herself showing indifference to others and hardly ever speaking; she now tells you she is intending suicide;

(iii) your elderly patient is living in conditions of increasing squalor; you are concerned for his health and safety; he has no relatives living nearby; he seems unable to fend for himself yet he clearly wants to stay where he is.

(a) What legal duties, if any, do you as a community health practitioner, have in these circumstances?
(b) What agencies are principally involved in dealing with these matters and what powers do they have?

Points to consider:

1(a) What offences, if any, are committed in respect of failing to report suspicions of crime?

1(b) Prevention of Terrorism Act 1989.

2(i) Social work departments and the Children Act 1989.

2(ii) Approved social workers and the Mental Health Act 1983.

2(iii) Social work departments, the community physician, s. 47 of the National Assistance Act 1948.

References and further reading

Employment law and industrial injury benefits

Encyclopedia of Health and Safety at Work in Law and Practice 1962. London: Sweet & Maxwell and W. Green & Son. (Updated loose leaf.)
Encyclopaedia of Labour Relations Law. London: Sweet & Maxwell and W. Green & Son. (Updated loose leaf.)
Fredman, S. and Morris, S. (1989) *The State as Employer: Labour Law in the Public Sector*. London: Mansell.
Ogus, A. and Barendt, E. (1988) *The Law of Social Security*. Butterworths.
Smith, I. T. and Wood, J. C. (1989) *Industrial Law*, 4th edn. London: Butterworths.

Tort liability – including negligence, occupiers' liability, animals

Andrews, A. P. (1991) Legal aspects in physiotherapy. In Jones, R. J. (ed) *Management in Physiotherapy*. Oxford: Radcliffe Medical Press.
Brazier, M. (1988) *Street on Torts*. 8th edn. London: Butterworths.
Buckley, R. A. (1988) *The Modern Law of Negligence*. London: Butterworths.
Clerk and Lindsell on Torts (1989). London: Sweet & Maxwell.
Jackson, R. and Powell, J. (1987) *Professional Negligence*, 2nd edn. London: Sweet & Maxwell.
Percy, R. (1990) *Charlesworth and Percy on Negligence*, 8th edn.
Powers, M. J. and Harris, N. H. (1990) *Medical Negligence*. London: Butterworths.

Involvement of Social Services Departments

Vernon, S. (1990) *Social Work and the Law*. London: Butterworths.
Brayne, H. and Martin, G. (1990) *Law for Social Workers*. London: Blackstone Press.

Cases

General Cleaning Contractors Ltd 1953 – *General Cleaning Contractors Ltd* v. *Christmas* [1953] AC 180.
Harris 1953 – *Harris* v. *Bright's Asphalt Contractors Ltd* 1953 1 All ER 395 Slade J.
McCloskey 1983 – *McCloskey* v. *Western Health and Social Services Board* 1983 4 NIJB CA.
Smith 1959 – *Smith* v. *Austin Lifts Co* [1959] 1 All ER 81.
Wilson 1958 – *Wilson* v. *Tyneside Window Cleaning Co* [1958] 2 QB 110.
Wyatt 1977 – *R* v. *Hillingdon A.H.A. ex parte Wyatt [1977]*.

Some useful addresses

Criminal Injuries Compensation Board, Blythswood House, 200 West Regent Street, Glasgow G2 4SW. (041-221 0945.)

Health and Safety Executive, Information Centre, Baynards House, 1 Chepstow Place, London W2 4TF. (071-243 6384.)

Health Visitors Association, 50 Southwark Street, London SE1 1UN. (071-378 7255.)

Chapter 5

Psychological issues

Sandra Horn

Introduction

In her introductory chapter to the book designed for physiotherapists from the 'Psychology for Professional Groups' series, Naomi Dunkin writes of the aim 'to develop a fuller understanding of human life, to identify human problems and to discover ways of reducing them as we find them'. All of us in the health care professions share that broad set of aims, but of necessity can only focus on those problems which fall within our own areas of expertise. One of the great benefits of working in the field of rehabilitation, however, is that one can be part of a team of people with common aims, and areas of expert knowledge which overlap and complement each other. Psychologists and physiotherapists share the desire to look beyond the immediate needs and emotional status of the rehabilitation client. They must look to the body of relevant literature, so that their skills as listeners, effective social interactors and therapists are sharpened by scientifically-based knowledge.

The following chapter contains a brief overview of some of the key social and clinical issues on which psychology has a bearing in community care. Included are psychological factors in ageing, sexuality, pain, grief and adaptive mechanisms in disability.

Ageing

This section explores some psychological factors in ageing. Mention will also be made of biological and social aspects of ageing, as they have a significant effect on attitudes, beliefs and psychological functioning.

What does ageing mean?

Ageing is a lifelong process of change and development. A baby ages to become a toddler; that is a process watched over with joy and hope by those concerned with the child. A difficult teenager might be exhorted to 'grow up'. That implies the expectation of improvement with ageing. It is only when it is applied to the later years that ageing has a negative connotation.

From the viewpoint of the person undergoing late-life ageing, the changes associated with it may be positive or neutral as well as negative.

Exercise

- Think back 10 years in your own life. In what ways have you changed since then?
- How many of the changes you have identified are positive from your point of view? Neutral? Negative?

He's wonderful for his age

Our society tends to group people by chronological age, as if everyone is at the same stage of development at x years old. Children go to school at five and leave at 16 or 18, ready or not. Adults retire at 65, ready or not. This artificial emphasis on dates obscures the fact that there is enormous variability among individuals at any age. This variability tends to increase rather than decrease with advancing age.

For large groups of people, averaged-out results from tests or surveys will show changes related to chronological age, but it is important to remember that each individual ages at a unique and variable pace.

Exercise

- Identify a small group of people, well known to you, who are of the same chronological age. Are they all at the same stage of age-development?
- How good are you at guessing other people's age? On what do you base your guesses?

What does old mean?

We are faced with a situation in which an increasing proportion of the population will be elderly. This does not mean that they will be ill or frail. However, there is a tendency for biological old age to be associated with changes which may affect health, directly or indirectly.

Elderly people have a decreased capacity for recovering from injury of illness as quickly or completely as they did when they were young.

There are changes in sensation associated with old age. Studies have shown that vision and hearing become less efficient. Stimuli are detected and discriminated less readily. Some clinical studies have suggested that these changes also affect taste, smell, touch and bodily sensations. The net result is that there is less information coming from the environment, and it is of reduced quality. Factors such as these tend to increase vulnerability to diseases and accidents. Uncorrected visual or hearing defects may be a factor in accidents. Decreased body sensation may allow disease to advance undetected. It has been suggested that a poor sense of taste and smell may be a contributory element in the inadequate diet of some old people (together with low income).

Two things are important here:

- These findings will be subject to wide individual variations.
- If the expectation is that these difficulties are inevitable (what can you expect at my age?), people may be deterred from seeking the help that is available.

Other changes associated with biological ageing include:

- loss of muscle power and elasticity of tissue, greying and thinning hair;
- the basal metabolic rate slows down.

These changes are normal, but can predispose the elderly person to a variety of health problems. Some of these problems may be psychological as the person struggles to adapt to unwelcome changes, such as having less energy and physical strength, or developing a typically elderly appearance.

There are also social changes associated with ageing, which may or may not be welcomed by the person experiencing them. Retirement from work can, for example, take away a sense of worth, as well as robbing the individual of a focus to the day, a social group and a decent income.

Children grow up and leave home, so that the role of parent changes and the immediate family circle shrinks. Further losses of social contact may be caused by bereavement.

Society also ascribes roles to its members; some of these are based on age. Grandad, pensioner, retired person, are examples of such

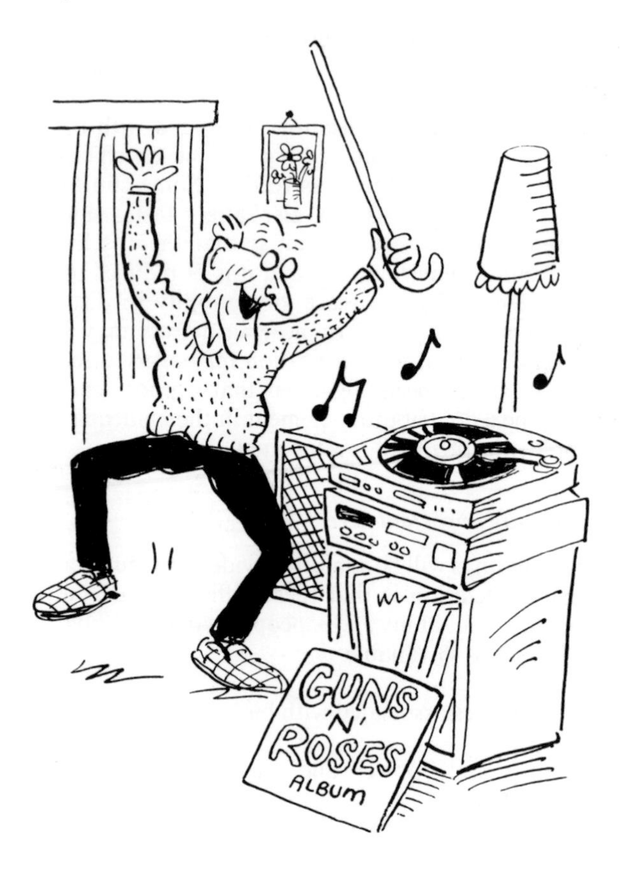

roles. They carry with them expectations about a variety of things such as physical appearance (including clothing, use of make-up, colour of hair) and behaviour. Old people are not expected to stay out late at the disco, play football, wear trendy clothes, flirt. They are expected to prefer sedentary hobbies such as watching television or knitting, or gentle exercise like walking. Anyone challenging these expectations may be made to feel odd.

Social and biological factors can have powerful psychological effects.

Exercise

- When you are old, how might your usual patterns of behaviour change?
- Why?
- How do you feel about it?

Psychological changes

Intellectual changes

In *Ageing and Society* Peter Coleman (1990) has pointed out that a marked bias exists in research into intellectual factors in old age. Studies have been directed almost exclusively towards those functions which decline. There has been little or no interest in those attributes of the individual which do not show deterioration.

In documenting the main findings of research into intellectual capacity and old age, two things should be borne in mind:

- The accumulated experience, wisdom and expertise, which may be hard to measure formally, but which has a considerable part to play in the mental life of the elderly person.
- The enormous variability which exists between people.

However, with advancing age, certain difficulties do become apparent:

- Stresses such as those caused by working against the clock, or by fear of failure, have an adverse effect on the elderly in problem-solving tasks. They tend to make more errors and proceed more slowly if pressured.
- Older people tend to opt for accuracy rather than speed in completing tests if given the choice, and may spend excessive amounts of time in checking that they are right.
- In problem-solving tasks, older people have difficulty in sifting out information they do not need, and ignoring it.
- Decision-making is slower.
- Older people are less inclined to guess or take risks.
- Divided attention (between two tasks or activities) tends to cause a marked decline in efficiency.
- Thinking may be rigid, so that old familiar ways may be adhered to when they are no longer appropriate.
- Memory for relatively meaningless information tends to be poor.
- Events tend to be recalled in general terms; unique or specific details are often 'lost'.
- Recall of memory test items after a short delay tends to be poor in the elderly, but recognition of the items is less so, suggesting that the problem is not so much one of storage, but retrieval.

It is apparent from this list that such things as learning and problem-solving can be assisted in the elderly if the material is presented in a meaningful and organised way, and self-pacing is permitted.

Yesavage and Jacob (1984) have shown that anxiety interferes with performance on attentional and memory tasks in the elderly, but relaxation training reduces the interference and improves recall.

Wilson (1989) has shown that the recall of health service information can be enhanced by the use of simple language rather than jargon, combined with categorising the material. Her study was carried out on a young sample, but Twining (1988) has also shown that encouraging the elderly to adopt strategies such as grouping things they need to remember into categories, can be beneficial.

Example

About the pain in your knee. First, I'm going to tell you what is causing it. Second, I'll tell you about when and how to rest it. Third, when to exercise, and how. Fourth, I'll explain about your tablets.

Exercise

Continue with the example given above and draw up a treatment plan for an elderly client with an arthritic knee, using simple language and categorisation. Bear in mind the finding that recognition memory is better than recall in the elderly.

Resource

'Managing Your Memory' contains a number of simple and clear ideas to help those with everyday memory problems. Contact Dr N. Kapur, Memory Aids Unit, Wessex Neurological Centre, Southampton General Hospital, Southampton SO9 4XY.

Personality

It has been suggested that there are certain changes in personality associated with old age:

- Increased passivity.
- Less expression of emotion.
- Increased conservatism.

- A tendency to introversion – preoccupation with the self and inner concerns rather than the outer world.

It is, however, hard to separate out these characteristics from the social and biological changes that old age brings. If old age means that fewer social opportunities and demands are made, many of these so-called 'personality changes' may be imposed from outside. Perhaps if the level of stimulation from the environment dropped, all of us would by necessity become more inner-directed.

Studies which have looked at ageing from a longitudinal viewpoint have tended to show that people remain very much as they have always been, with the same basic characteristics, habits, ways of coping. Interests and activities, where the opportunities for them are present, also tend to remain stable.

Some values and interests may in fact grow stronger when there is more time to give them.

As with intellectual abilities, any marked change in personality in old age should be a cause for alarm, as it may herald the onset of a condition such as dementia or depression.

Exercise

- List 10 things you consider to be abiding characteristics of yours.
- Can you remember a time when you were different? If so, what was it that made you change?

Pathological psychological changes in old age

The following is an account of the main features of some common disorders associated with old age. It does not include the psychotic states, for an account of which the reader is referred to Bromley (1966).

1. Dementia

The changes in intellectual ability mentioned above tend to happen gradually. Any marked or rapid change in mental functioning, mood or behaviour in an elderly person should always be a cause of concern.

Such dramatic change could indicate the onset or worsening of a physical problem such as cardiac inefficiency, or a toxic or infective state, or the beginning of clinical depression. On the other hand, it could be the first sign of one of the chronic brain disorders known as dementia.

Investigation of the health status of the client is of the utmost importance as the physical condition or the depression may be treatable.

At the time of writing primary dementia is not treatable, although some of its manifestations, such as agitation, can be ameliorated with drugs.

Some forms of dementia have a known cause, such as arteriosclerosis or chronic alcoholism. Some are familial. Others, such as Alzheimer's disease, show characteristic changes in brain tissue but a precise cause has yet to be identified.

Bromley (1966) has described the psychological effects of these chronic brain disorders as follows:

- Loss of judgement and intellectual powers.
- Failure of memory.
- Disorientation in time and place.

As the condition progresses (the rate and progress will be variable), other changes may be added to the list:

- Mood may be flattened, or agitated and anxious, volatile, or depressed.
- Energy level may drop markedly.
- Personal habits may decline.
- Sleep may be disturbed.

Some types of dementia may be accompanied by severe psychiatric disturbances such as paranoia, depression, delusions and hallucinations. Again, diagnosis is of primary importance so that such things as toxic confusional states may be excluded.

2. Depression

Depression is more common in the elderly than in any other age group. Some of the reasons for its increased prevalence may be social:

- Retirement, with its associated loss of daily contact with a social group, loss of purpose and focus, loss of job status and loss of income.
- It also leads to increased leisure time, which can be positive, but which can also be a problem if poor health or low income

prevent access to leisure opportunities. Time may lie heavily on the hands.

- Family groups change as children grow up and move away.
- Losses through bereavement tend to increase with increased age.
- The grief of bereavement may be compounded by loneliness and relative social isolation.
- There may be a need to relocate to a new neighbourhood or to smaller living accommodation, or to a residential home with care assistance. Moves such as these bring with them a variety of losses.

Physical changes may also contribute to the onset of depression:

- Disease or illness causing pain or discomfort, or the need for help with intimate body functions so that privacy and dignity are compromised, or resulting in problems with mobility, or increased dependence.
- Infectious diseases, not necessarily serious, but resulting in lowered mood or energy – 'post-viral syndrome'.
- A period of disruption such as that caused by an operation or other reasons for a stay in hospital.
- A problem directly affecting the brain, such as stroke or head injury.
- Malnutrition.

Psychological factors are also important:

- The need for adjustment to unwelcome change.
- Anxiety related to fears for the future, including fear of impending terminal illness or death.
- A sense of worthlessness with the loss of social roles.

Depression is more than a feeling of sadness and tearfulness. Although these things may be the obvious and outward signs of the condition, they are not always present in a depressed person.

Symptoms of depression may include the following:

- Disturbed sleep.
- Poor appetite.
- Apathy.
- Self-neglect.
- Anxiety.
- Pessimism.
- Distractedness, leading to impaired memory function.

- Disturbance of thinking; often, ideas of persecution or of being punished.

It will be seen from this list that there is often a similarity between the symptoms of depression and those of dementia. Expert assessment is of the utmost importance, as depression is usually treatable, initially with drugs, or ECT in certain cases. Counselling or psychotherapy may also be important once recovery has progressed to the point where the client is able to benefit. Planning for the future so as to prevent recurrences is also crucial. The psychogeriatric team is the appropriate agency from which to obtain expert help in diagnosis, treatment and management.

Psychological factors in disability

When a disease or a disorder fails to recover completely, and the consequences of it are likely to be long lasting or permanent, there is a need to adjust to the fact that life will be different. Sometimes, a period of grieving is experienced as part of that adjustment. As Anderson and Bury (1988) have pointed out, the experience of chronic illness is a process of change over time; of resolution and renegotiation of roles and relationships. This highlights the fact that disability happens not just to the individual, but to the family and close others. All of them will be affected by the need for change and adjustment in the disabled individual. The Social Readjustment Rating Scale of Holmes and Rahe (1967), developed to assess the degree of change needed to cope with a variety of life events, shows high ratings for 'major personal injury or illness' and 'major change in health or behaviour of a family member'.

The issues discussed in this chapter apply to the disabled person and his/her close others equally.

Many factors will influence, for better or worse, that process of adjustment. Some factors arise from the disorder, such as:

- Severity.
- Onset (gradual, sudden, traumatic).
- Progression (static from onset, tending to improve somewhat, tending to deteriorate).
- Course (predictable, unpredictable).
- Character (painful, disfiguring, leading to dependence).
- Focus (special senses, limbs, brain, and thus behaviour, emotions, mental abilities, personality; other vital organs, body chemistry. May also affect brain functions).

Particular difficulties in adjustment are caused when the disorder affects brain function. The capacity to learn and adapt may be impaired, and personality and behaviour changed.

Pain can also affect adaptation. Obvious disfigurement, which immediately marks the sufferer out as 'different', can result in social isolation. The struggle to deal with other people's discomfort can sometimes be too much to bear. Moves towards integrating everyone into the community, and efforts to make the environment user-friendly for all (and therefore not needing special provisions for disabled people), are relatively new, and have been spearheaded by disabled groups and farsighted professionals. These changes are gathering momentum, and should at the very least break down the social barriers caused by unfamiliarity.

Other factors are social, such as:

- Support of family and friends.
- Work prospects.
- Leisure prospects.
- Living arrangements.
- Financial implications.
- Environmental barriers to integration.
- Acceptance by the community.
- Stage of the life-cycle (adolescent, young parent, retired).

Finally, there are the psychological attributes of the person with the disorder, such as:

- Coping style.
- Sense of self-worth.
- Confidence.
- Beliefs, values, attitudes.
- Practical intelligence.
- Emotional resources.

Combinations of these factors will help to determine the level of adjustment to the disorder. Wood (1980) has produced a model showing the steps from the initial disorder through impairment and disability to handicap:

Disease or disorder

Impairment

The individual becomes aware that he or she is unhealthy or

unusual. Impairment relates to abnormalities of body structure or appearance, and organ or system function.

Impairment represents disturbance at the organ level.

Disability

Disability reflects the consequences of impairments in terms of the performance of activities; it represents disturbances at the level of the person.

Handicap

The individual is placed at a disadvantage relative to others. Handicap is a social concept, reflecting an adverse value placed on an individual's performance or status when these are compromised by impairments or disabilities.

Coping with disability; initial needs

Human beings are adaptable; they tend to explore and try to make sense of any new situation, and then behave so that they can at least survive in it, and at most, capitalise on it.

Exploration is aimed at getting essential information. The new situation must be understood.

- ***There is a need for education and advice***

When we try to make sense of a new situation, we often do so by comparing it with something from past experience, or talking about it with people who will listen carefully and try to understand. As Hasler (1985) says, 'A supportive enabling strategy demands an understanding of the ideas, concerns and expectations of patients.'

- ***There is a need for discussion***

The mass of information coming in a new situation needs to be organised so that problems can be defined and given priorities according to urgency.

This will facilitate goal-setting and action plans. Egan (1986) has suggested a problem-management approach as an effective way of assisting change.

- ***There is a need for skilled help***

Coping with disability; the individual

Unless the disability to be faced is one which has impaired the individual's capacity for thinking, planning and organising, the idea of self-responsibility will be crucial in coping. Rotter (1966) has suggested that the locus of control is an important determinant of behaviour. That is, whether someone tends to believe that events are influenced more by luck or powerful others (external locus of control) or by oneself (internal locus of control). Other authors have investigated this theory in a variety of health-care settings, including the treatment of stuttering (Craig *et al.* 1984) and stroke and wrist fracture (Partridge and Johnson 1989). These studies have tended to show a relationship between locus of control as measured by questionnaire, and outcome. That is, that a greater belief in personal control (greater internality) is predictive of a faster and more complete recovery. There is also the suggestion that in some people the locus changes as recovery takes place, from external to internal, and they are less likely to relapse than those who remain with an external locus.

These results beg the question of whether locus of control is a relatively stable trait of personality, or can be modified by experience. In the early stages of coping with disability, anyone might be overwhelmed with a sense of events being beyond their control; this is a normal response to crisis. What is needed is to identify the process necessary to change the perceived locus from external to internal.

Other approaches to the problem of people feeling unable to take responsibility for themselves have been described by Schiff (1975):

- Passivity.

and by Seligman (1975):

- Learned helplessness.

Ellis (1974) and Parry (1990) have discussed self-talk of a negative or disabling kind. This behaviour will be readily recognised by most people. It consists of an internal dialogue with statements such as 'I can't. I won't be able to cope. I must be going mad. My life is ruined.'

Again, this is a common response to an overwhelming change.

Parry (1990) and Hopson (1981) both recommend the conscious adoption of positive self-talk to counteract its effects – for example, 'I can come through this. I've been in bad situations before and it turned out all right. I'll take this one a bit at a time.'

Other methods of facilitating coping and self-directed change are described below.

Hopson (1981) and his colleagues have developed a questionnaire to help people identify the coping skills they already possess, as well as gaps in their skills or understanding, which can then be addressed in workshops.

The questionnaire covers areas such as:

- Knowing yourself.
- Knowing your new situation.
- Knowing other people who can help.
- Learning from the past.
- Looking after yourself.
- Letting go of the past.
- Setting goals and making action plans.
- Looking for gains you have made.

Egan (1986) has suggested that people's sense of self-efficacy can be strengthened in four ways:

- Success. If people can see that their actions produce results, even in small ways, they will be encouraged to go on and try something more difficult.
- Modelling. Seeing others behaving successfully in something they themselves want to do will encourage them to try.
- Encouragement. Other people encouraging and challenging them and supporting their efforts.
- Reducing fear and anxiety. Fear of failure may mean that an individual will not attempt something. Anything which reduces that fear will enhance self-efficacy.

Exercise

Outline a programme of treatment to encourage a joint-protection approach to housework in someone with rheumatoid arthritis, bearing Egan's four points in mind.

Grieving

Grief is more than a sense of deep sorrow associated with loss. Colin Murray Parkes (1975) describes it as an emotional and behavioural reaction set in chain when a love-tie is broken. We usually think of grieving in association with bereavement; that is, loss by death.

However, there are less obvious losses which can result in grief. Retirement, moving house, children growing up and leaving, loss of a body function or part of one's body; all these things and many others can cause a period of grieving.

Having the diagnosis of a chronic or life-threatening illness confirmed may also provoke a grief reaction. Where the course of the condition is unpredictable, as in multiple sclerosis, there is no one episode or loss to act as a focus, so grief may not resolve readily, and may be ever-present in the background, giving rise to acute surges of mourning from time to time. It is important that this is recognised and assisted by expert counsellors.

In the following account, loss by death is referred to, but the salient points refer to grief triggered by any kind of significant loss.

Does grief follow a set of stages?

In an attempt to produce a systematic picture of grief, some theorists have proposed that there is a series of stages or steps that the bereaved person goes through – a 'process'. For example:

- Numbness, shock.
- Denial.
- Anger.
- Depression, despair.
- Adaptation.

While it is true that people go through different phases as they grieve, it is a mistake to suppose that there is an orderly progression from one to another, or that everyone goes through all of the same phases.

Certain feelings do tend to occur in the course of grieving, such as sadness and yearning, guilt and self-reproach, anger, anxiety. C. S. Lewis (1961) wrote that he had never realised how much grief would feel like fear. Odd sensations like butterflies in the stomach or a tight throat may be experienced in the early stages. These are like fear, and are caused by the same mechanism, the 'fight or flight' syndrome we experience when we are under threat. To have lost, forever, an important part of one's life is threatening.

Fatigue, helplessness and loneliness are also common. The grieving person is struggling with an overwhelming change, so a distressing mixture of emotions is not surprising. People may also behave in an uncharacteristic way, and become absent-minded, have disturbances of sleep and appetite, become withdrawn. They may have vivid dreams, in which the loss has not taken place, and wake up unable to tell truth from dreaming for a moment; they may hear the voice of the lost one, or 'see' them in the street; they may have an overwhelming sense of the presence of one who has died.

All these things may occur frequently in the early stages after loss, and are part of the struggle to adapt to a new and perhaps unwelcome life, and accept that the old familiar one has gone. They tend to become less frequent as time goes on, but may go on erupting from time to time over a long period of months.

However:

- Each person will be unique in their pattern of reactions.
- The list of things mentioned is not exhaustive, nor is it a prescription for grief.

Exercise

Think back to a loss of any kind which you have suffered. List all the feelings associated with it. How long do you think they took to resolve?

Some determinants of grief

Certain factors help to determine the intensity and length of grief after bereavement:

- The relationship to the one who has died – parent, child, spouse.
- The closeness of the attachment.
- Ambivalence in the relationship – can make grief complicated.
- The mode of death – sudden; traumatic; witnessed by the bereaved; suicide; expected; time to prepare.
- The personality of the bereaved one, and the presence of other problems at the time, such as illness.
- The availability of good social support.
- What the bereavement means in terms of disruption to life – will it lead to loss of home, loss of income, social isolation?

Beverley Raphael (1984) identified risk-factors in a group of widows:

- non-supportive social network;
- traumatic circumstances of death;
- ambivalent marital relationship;
- concurrent life-crisis, such as illness.

In her study, the widows were divided into two groups. One group received regular support and were encouraged to express their grief. The other group received no intervention. At follow-up, the unsupported group showed high incidences of such problems as sleeplessness, back pain, swollen joints, weight loss, rheumatism, poor appetite, panic attacks and sweating. They made more visits to the doctor, and increased smoking, drinking and tablet taking. They tended to complain of excessive tiredness, depression and decreased work capacity.

As Raphael has pointed out, the cost of providing regular support is minimal, especially when it is compared to the cost (human and economic) of not providing that support.

A very real difficulty in providing support for the bereaved is knowing what to do and what to say. Bereaved people often complain that others avoid them, and it is frequently because finding the right words is a problem.

Davidovitz and Myrick (1984) interviewed people who had experienced a death in their family, and asked them what sort of comments from others they had found helpful or not helpful.

Unhelpful	***Helpful***
He (God) had a purpose	Come and be with us now
It is God's will	You're being very strong
Be thankful you have another son	It's OK to be angry at God
I know how you feel	It must be hard to accept
Time makes it easier	That must be painful for you
You shouldn't question God's will	You must have been very close
You have to keep on going	Tell me how you're feeling
You have to get on with life	How can I be of help?
It's inevitable	Let's spend time together
You're not the only one who suffers	Go ahead and grieve
That's over now, let's not dwell on it	People really cared for him
The living must go on	I'm praying for you
She has led a full life	

On the unhelpful side, the comments prescribe remedies and give instructions. On the helpful side, they express sympathy and solidarity, and ask what help is needed.

We cannot cure another's grief, but we may lessen the burden by sharing it. Nor can we speed up someone else's mourning by exhorting them to cheer up or by telling them it is time they were over it. The best kind of support is uncritical and kindly.

Abnormal grief

Raphael and others have identified risk factors which tend to complicate and prolong grief. However, patterns of grieving vary, so how can an abnormal grief, which will need professional intervention, be recognised?

Parkes has suggested two watchpoints:

- Chronic intense grief which does not seem to change. He mentions people who remained preoccupied with thoughts of the dead person, pining intensely and severely distressed by any reminder of them, long after the initial weeks or months.
- Delayed reaction. People who had not shown any reaction initially, and had gone on behaving as if nothing had happened, and had then suddenly after some days begun to grieve, were also at risk of going on to need professional help.

Worden (1988) describes two other pathological reactions:

- Exaggerated grief.
- Masked grief, which appears in the form of a physical symptom or aberrant behaviour.

These are grief reactions complicated by something unresolved. They can often be helped by counselling or grief therapy.

The end of mourning

Worden has suggested that there are four tasks of mourning:

1. To accept the reality of the loss.
2. To experience the pain of grief.
3. To adjust to an environment in which the deceased is missing.
4. To withdraw emotional energy and invest it in another relationship.

Not everyone will be able to accomplish all of the tasks. Elderly people who have lost a spouse, for example, may not be able to adjust fully, and may never go on to invest in another relationship.

Most people will accomplish the tasks of grief naturally, or with the assistance of grief counsellors or grief therapists. They will reach a stage of acceptance and adjustment, be able to form satisfactory new relationships and be able to think of their lost one without pain.

These are large tasks, and they will not usually be accomplished quickly.

Pain

A simple view of pain is that it is an unpleasant sensation experienced when the body is injured or afflicted by some kinds of disease.

The experience of pain is:

- Unpleasant.
- Urgent.
- Hard to ignore.

It causes arousal in the sympathetic nervous system, in the same way that fear and anger do. For example:

- Heart-rate and respiration rate increase.
- Blood-pressure is raised.

These changes help to prepare the body for rapid action. The arousal of the sympathetic nervous system is associated with a strong emotional reaction, which helps to stamp the situation in which the pain is occurring, into the memory. Too close an encounter with a sharp knife or a hot iron in the future will bring the unpleasant memory flooding back; this facilitates the learning of avoidance behaviour.

Pain helps us to adapt our behaviour so as to increase our chances of survival.

This simple view of pain of the acute type is, however, far from the whole story. The relationship between pain and tissue damage is complex. Consider the following examples:

- Referred pain (the damage is in one place, the pain in another).
- Trigger zone (stimulating one area causes pain somewhere else).
- Phantom pain (pain experienced in a limb after amputation).
- Silent pathological changes (damage in the absence of pain).
- Chronic pain (continuing pain outliving its cause, or after healing appears to be complete, or in the absence of a visible lesion).

These examples demonstrate that there is no fixed relationship between tissue damage and pain.

The experience of pain is modified by a range of factors, both internal and external to the sufferer.

Measuring pain

In the laboratory, it is possible to demonstrate a relationship between the intensity of a stimulus (heat, cold, electric shock, pressure) and perceived pain. Pain threshold, the point at which the subject says the stimulus hurts, can be shown, as well as pain tolerance, which is the point at which the subject requests termination of the stimulus because it is unbearable.

- Pain intensity is estimated from what the subject says.
- Pain tolerance is estimated from observing the subject's behaviour.

These two points are important because, in or out of the laboratory, they are the only ways of estimating someone else's pain.

There are pain-measurement scales; here are examples of the types most commonly used:

Descriptive scale

- No pain.
- Mild pain.
- Moderate pain.
- Severe pain.
- Extreme pain.

Place a tick by the statement which best describes the amount of pain you are feeling now.

Visual analogue scale

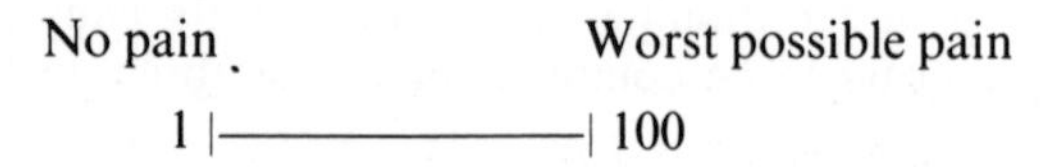

Make a mark on the line to show the amount of pain you are feeling now.

Functional scale

- Walking causes me no pain.
- Walking causes me some pain.
- Walking causes me severe pain.
- Walking is impossible because of pain.

Tick the statement which best describes how your pain affects your walking.

Scales suitable for children, such as the Pain Thermometer, where the child is asked to colour in a column with the height corresponding to the amount of pain they feel, or Fear Faces, in which the child selects from a series of facial expressions the one closest to their feelings, have also been developed (Katz *et al.* 1982a,b).

There are also methods using observation of pain behaviour, where the frequency of such things as groaning or crying, mentioning the pain, or asking for pain-relieving drugs, is recorded.

It is important to remember that the scores on all these measures have no absolute values. Putting numbers on them gives a rough estimate of whether the pain is better or worse under certain conditions for individual people, but the numbers are still based on subjective estimates.

Pain modifiers

Melzack (1973) proposed the gate control theory of pain. In essence, the theory is that the perception of pain is an interaction between input from 'pain fibres' in the peripheral nervous system, and central (brain) factors.

- The action of the pain fibres can be changed by input from the surrounding nerve endings. A simple example is that when we knock a limb on something hard, we can modify the pain by rubbing the surrounding area. The stimulation of the nerve endings produced by rubbing the skin has the effect of dulling the pain. The stimuli appear to compete, and the effect of lots of other sensory nerve endings being activated at once, by rubbing the skin, is to overwhelm the input from pain fibres.

It may be that the pain reduction produced by TENS (transcutaneous electrical nerve stimulation) works in the same way.

- The perception of pain is also heavily influenced by input from the brain. The input is not only from the action of nerves and neuro-chemicals such as endorphins, psychological factors play an important part. They include the following:

- learning
- expectation and belief
- meaning
- context
- emotions, such as fear
- sense of control.

We do not have to learn to feel pain, but there is an element of learning in our reaction to pain. A small child often looks at its mother if it falls over, as if waiting for her reaction before knowing how to react itself. If mother is distressed, the child cries. If mother calmly says 'Whoops-a-daisy, up you get', the child is more likely to think there is nothing to worry about, and go on playing.

Distress increases pain. Therefore, if we learn to be distressed when we have a minor bump, we influence our perception of pain.

The role of expectation in pain is amply illustrated by the marked distress shown by burned children who have to undergo frequent painful procedures as part of their treatment. It might be expected that they would adapt as the days go by, but if anything, their distress increases. Presumably, as soon as they see the clinic room in which the treatment is carried out, the memory of the pain associated with it produces the expectation of further pain. This leads to fear, and fear increases pain.

Some researchers (Elliott and Olson 1983; Kelly *et al.* 1984) have demonstrated the effectiveness of techniques such as attention–distraction (using cartoons), relaxation breathing, imagery and reinterpreting the context of the pain, on the distress shown by burned children. It appears that if the association between pain and the situation can be broken by the use of these interventions, children can learn to adapt, and appear to feel less pain.

The meaning of pain will exert a powerful influence over its perception. Does it mean cancer? Does it mean a recurrence of an old familiar problem which tends to last a short time and then go away, and which is not sinister? Does it mean I can have a day off school? Does it mean that healing is taking place? Does it mean I am free from a boring and repetitive duty I have never liked? Does it mean the end of my sporting career? These and many other meanings attached to pain will colour how it is perceived.

The context in which pain occurs is also important. If an old lady on her own at home receives a blow on the shin of exactly the same force as one delivered to the shin of a young footballer about to shoot for goal, they not only react differently, but they are likely to feel different degrees of pain. The footballer's mind is powerfully distracted by events around him and the overriding importance of winning the game. The old lady is alone with her pain and her worry about how much damage she has done.

Emotions such as fear, already mentioned here, modify pain. Fear and anxiety are associated with activation of the sympathetic nervous system, in which a heightened awareness (part of the 'fight or flight' reaction to danger) increases the experience of pain.

A sense of control can diminish pain. Egbert *et al.* (1964) have shown that patients who received detailed instructions about what to expect and how to deal with it, after major surgery, reported less pain than those who did not. Beales (1983) recommends involving the sufferer in the therapy as a means of increasing a sense of control.

Chronic pain

When pain becomes chronic, it retains the characteristics of acute pain. That is, it is unpleasant, urgent, hard to ignore, and it causes activation of the sympathetic nervous system. In chronic, as in any pain, the sufferer tends to behave so as to try to reduce the intensity of the experience. This is adaptive behaviour.

Resting, avoiding activities which bring on the pain or make it worse, and taking medicine are common ways in which acute pain may be reduced. Unfortunately, they may compound the problem in chronic pain, in the following ways:

- Resting and avoiding daily tasks can leave long stretches of the day unoccupied. Pain has an all-pervasive quality. It is hard to ignore, and will tend to dominate the thinking of a sufferer who has nothing else to distract them.
- Pain-killing drugs, especially strong drugs, work by depressing the nervous system. They may produce clouding of consciousness, so that clear thinking is impossible; they may cause depressed mood and apathy; they frequently have side-effects such as constipation; the body tends to adapt to them, so that more drugs are needed to produce the same effect as time goes on.

These are not neurotic behaviours, but inappropriate attempts to manage the pain. They tend to lead to long periods of inactivity, in which the pain dominates thinking because of its urgency and the fact that it is hard to ignore. The unpleasantness of the pain, and its emotional tone, are depressing. Lowered mood may be further depressed by the action of strong pain-killers, and a growing sense of helplessness and dependency.

Some victims begin by using the feelings of urgency to try to 'fight' the pain. They may throw themselves into bursts of physical activity, which come to an abrupt end when the pain becomes severe. They will then take medication and rest, but with little hope of a good response.

These two patterns of behaviour, passivity and alternating activity/passivity, are common responses to chronic pain. They may produce secondary gains:

- They allow the pain sufferer to avoid things they would rather not do.
- They involve family and friends in caring for the sufferer.

In cases like these, motivation for changes in the pattern of behaviour may be low or absent. However, most chronic pain victims are unhappy with the turn their lives have taken, and would prefer to manage their pain constructively, if they could. For people such as these, there are an increasing number of pain management programmes available within the health service.

Fordyce *et al.* (1968) working in America, originated the idea of the pain management programme. In the UK, up and down the country, these programmes differ in details such as the length of time of treatment, and inpatient versus outpatient regimens, but they all have essential elements in common.

- The pain itself is not the focus of the programme. Treatment is aimed at the behaviour associated with the pain. For example, physiotherapy may be used to tone up muscles and improve fitness, but will not be targeted on the painful area.
- Painkilling medication is withdrawn. In some regimens, all medicine is given in the form of an elixir. A standard dose is given at set times during the day. Throughout the programme, the active drugs are reduced, but the amount of liquid stays constant, so that anxiety about drug reduction is avoided. Patients agree the regimen at the outset, and know that their drugs will be reduced, but they do not know by how much, or when.
- An increasing programme of paced daily activity is undertaken.
- Pacing of daily routine may be taught as a pain-avoiding technique (rather than excessive resting or cycles of under- and over-activity).

- Pain behaviour is ignored (i.e. not reinforced by gaining attention).
- Alternative methods of pain control are taught, such as deep muscular relaxation.
- Education is given about the nature of pain, how the chronic pain syndrome arises, and how it can be better managed.
- A close friend or relative (usually someone who lives with the patient) may be involved. This is to help other people who have become part of the pain behaviour cycle to change their ways too.
- There must be a commitment on the part of the patient, to enter fully into the programme, on the understanding that it is about management, not cure.

Many of the lessons learned from chronic pain programmes can be applied to conditions such as rheumatoid arthritis, as long as essential drug regimens are adhered to. The use of pacing, relaxation and education can all be used to enhance pain control.

Exercise

Think of the last time you were in pain. Was it mild, severe, brief, longlasting? How did you manage it? How successful was your strategy? How effective do you think it would have been in the long term?

Sexual behaviour

Even now, in the years following the so-called 'permissive society', there is ignorance about normal human sexual behaviour. This is, in part, because sexual behaviour is largely regarded as a private matter. The openness about sexual matters in literature, theatre and film productions has not necessarily become the norm in conversations between ordinary people. One source of difficulty is the language. Between technical terms and obscenity there is something of a gap; it is not easy to find widely acceptable and widely understood terminology.

For these, and no doubt other reasons, myths, rumours and half-truths abound. There are tales about ideal 'performance', for example, which may be publicly regarded as jokes, but which may at the same time cause private worries. What if they are true? How inadequate does that make me? If I don't know what normal is, how do I know if I am?

In addition to the language problem, and the natural reticence people may feel about discussing something they have been brought up to regard as private (and perhaps shameful), there is the fact that ideas of self-worth, masculinity and feminity may be bound up with perceived sexual adequacy. The mythology of sex can exert a strong influence, particularly on the young, who may be struggling to establish themselves as people capable of having an intimate relationship. Sex is commonly supposed to be both instinctive and easy. For very many people it is neither, but that is not part of the popular myth.

Another common belief is that sex can strengthen a relationship, bring couples close together emotionally, and resolve tension. While this is often true, particularly in a relationship that is good to start with, the other side of the coin is that sex can also sometimes be a potent source of tension and anxiety. Differences in needs and preferred behaviour between people can cause considerable anguish, especially if discussion of the problems is made difficult by shyness and the lack of an adequate language. Who knows what multitude of problems is glossed over by 'Not tonight. I've got a headache.'?

Exercise

How many euphemisms can you think of for sexual intercourse and the sex organs? You might like to compare lists with colleagues, to see what overlap there is, and what incidence of exclusive usage. Of all the jokes you know, what proportion of them is about sex? Why do we make jokes about sex?

Sexual problems

We do not know what the exact incidence of sexual difficulties is in the population. It would be a reasonable assumption that most people will experience problems at one time or another, since a wide variety of things have an influence on sexual behaviour, and in any relationship there are bound to be periods of mismatch between one person's needs and the other's. In the case of a long-term difficulty, some people may feel able to request help, others may suffer in silence through embarrassment, or ignorance about where to go for assistance, or because they think that the problem is just one of those things and cannot be helped.

The most common problem reported in men is premature ejaculation. That is, ejaculation happening before the partner can reach orgasm, and in extreme cases, before penetration. Impotence or failure of erection is the next most common.

The most commonly reported problem in women is failure of orgasm. Another is progressive lack of interest in sex, sometimes leading to aversion.

Men and women alike tend to have sexual problems because of psychological factors:

- Fear and anxiety.
- Depression.
- Attitudes and beliefs.
- Lack of knowledge about sexual functioning.
- Poor technique on the part of self or partner.

There are physical factors in sexual dysfunction too, although they are probably much less common. Some are well documented, such as impotence secondary to diabetes mellitus, or the effect of drugs such as beta-blockers. Problems such as these stand a better chance of receiving attention, since doctors and other health workers might be looking out for them.

Help is available in a variety of centres. Some health authorities run sexual dysfunction clinics; family planning clinics, organisations such as RELATE, and GPs will offer treatment or put people in touch with an appropriate agency. Most of the treatments are based around changing behaviour and expectations, and will usually expect to involve both partners.

Sex and disability

People disabled from birth, or by disease or accident, are not immune to sexual feelings and needs, and therefore not immune to sexual problems. They will be prone to all the difficulties already mentioned, and possibly some extra ones directly or indirectly associated with their condition.

There are, for example, conditions affecting the nervous system which can inhibit erection and/or ejaculation, and inhibit the increase in blood flow to the vagina and lubrication. They include:

- Multiple sclerosis.
- Diabetes mellitus.
- Spina bifida.
- Spinal injury (although erection may occur as a reflex).

Other conditions have an effect by restricting movement, including:

- Arthritis (also causes pain).
- Paralysis.
- Spasticity.

Some conditions require drug treatment which may cause impotence, including:

- Heart attack.
- Depression.
- Some forms of cancer.

Some conditions, such as sexual disinhibition or increased sexuality, sometimes seen after head injury or stroke, may need drug treatment or behavioural treatment aimed at decreasing the behaviour. In other cases, all sexual feeling and interest may be absent after brain injury.

Sometimes, fear of sexual activity is a problem, notably after such conditions as stroke or heart attack, where arousal might cause a recurrence.

Other conditions may inhibit sexual functioning because they involve mutilation or disturbances of body felt to be shameful, so that the victim withdraws from close contact. They include:

- Amputation.
- Mastectomy.
- Deformity.
- Scarring.
- Colostomy.
- Urinary incontinence.

Some solutions

Milton Diamond (1977) has made a crucial point about sexuality:

> For the able-bodied as well as the handicapped, we should do away with the myth which in essence states that the only satisfactory means of expressing oneself sexually and achieving satisfaction is with an erect penis in a well-lubricated vagina.

He further goes on to make the following points:

Anybody's sex life can be improved by

- Increased communication.
- Decreased guilt with anything mutually satisfying.
- Education and ease in dealing openly with sexual issues, so that expectations are more realistically in line with performance capabilities.

The sex researchers and therapists, Masters and Johnson, suggest that 'normal' is what is acceptable to both partners and does not involve damage (Masters and Johnson 1980). With these tenets in mind, it is clear that a wide variety of possibilities exists. Close loving physical contact leading to mutual pleasure can be achieved in a variety of postures, using any part of the body. Sex aids, such as lubricants, vibrators, energising rings (to aid erections), dildos and artificial vaginas are readily available, and can be valuable if both partners feel happy and relaxed in using them. Sex manuals are full of inventive ideas, and in Grieve's (1981) book there are drawings showing positions suitable for those with serious back problems. Some of them would also suit people with other physical difficulties involving pain or restricted movement.

For those people whose disability carries with it an element of fear or shame, or for the partners of those with abnormally

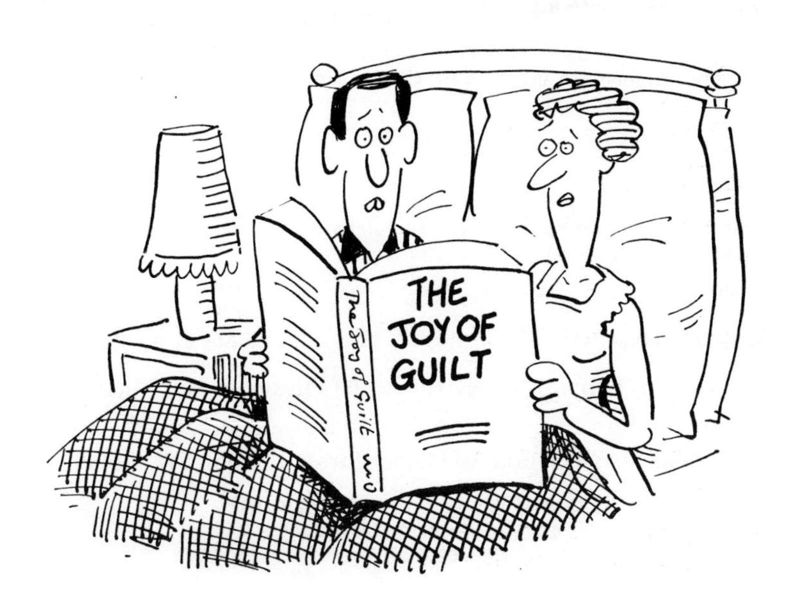

increased or decreased sexuality, support, counselling and information are crucial.

Guidelines are available about when to resume sexual activity after a heart attack, and how to cope with incontinence (Davies 1988).

Role of the professional

The health care professional should be able to deal with questions of sexuality. Not everyone is comfortable with the topic, and it is not necessary that they should be, but everyone should be aware that sexuality is a legitimate concern of clients, and should, at the least, be able to provide information on sources of help.

References

Ageing

Bromley, D. (1966) *The Psychology of Human Ageing*. London: Pelican.

Coleman P. (1990) Psychological ageing. In Bond, J. and Coleman, P., eds. *Ageing in Society*. pp. 62–88. London: Sage Publications.

Twining, C. (1988) *Helping Older People: a Psychological Approach*. Chichester: Wiley.

Wilson, B. (1989) Improving recall of Health Service information, *Clinical Rehabilitation*, **3**, 275–279.

Yesavage, J. A. and Jacob, R. (1984) Effects of relaxation and mnemonics on memory, attention and anxiety in the elderly, *Experimental Ageing Research*, **10** (4), 211–214.

Further reading

Windmill, V. (1990) *Ageing Today: a Positive Approach to Caring for Elderly People*. London: Edward Arnold.

Useful addresses

Age Concern, Bernard Sunley House, 60 Pitcairn Road, Mitcham, Surrey CR4 3LL.

Pre-retirement Association, 19 Undine Street, London SW17 8PP.

Help the Aged, St James' Walk, London EC1R 0BE.

Disability

Anderson, R. and Bury, M. (1988) *Living With Chronic Illness.* London: Unwin Hyman.
Craig, A. R. *et al.* (1984) A scale to measure locus of control of behaviour. *Br. J. Med. Psychol.,* **57,** 173–180.
Egan, G. (1986) *The Skilled Helper.* London: Brooks/Cole.
Ellis, A. (1974) *Disputing Irrational Beliefs (DIBS).* New York. Institute for Rational Living.
Hasler, J. C. (1985) The very stuff of general practice, *J. R. Coll. Gen. Practit.,* **35,** 121–1275.
Holmes, T. H. and Rahe, R. H. (1967) Methodological aspects of life events research, *J. Psychosom. Res.,* **27** (5), 341–352.
Hopson, B. (1981) Transition: understanding and managing personal change. In Griffiths, D. ed. *Psychology and Medicine.* London: BPS/Macmillan.
Parry, G. (1990) *Coping With Crises.* London: BPS/Routledge.
Partridge, C. and Johnson, M. (1989) Perceived control of recovery from physical disability: measurement and prediction, *Br. J. Clin. Psychol.,* **28,** 53–59.
Rotter J. B. (1966) Generalised expectancies for internal versus external control of reinforcement, *Psychological Monographs,* **80,** 1–28.
Schiff, J. L. (1975) Cathexis reader. In *Transactional Analysis Treatment of Psychosis.* New York: Harper and Row.
Seligman, M. E. P. (1975) *Helplessness: on Depression, Development, and Death.* San Francisco: Freeman.
Wood, P. H. N. (1980) The language of disablement: a glossary relating to disease and its consequences, *Int. Rehabil. Med.,* **2,** 86–92.

Recommended reading

Goodwill, C. J. and Chamberlain, M. A. (eds) (1988) *Rehabilitation of the Physically Disabled Adult.* London: Croom Helm.

Grieving

Davidovitz, M. and Myrick, R. D. (1984) Responding to the bereaved: an analysis of helping statements, *Death Education,* **8,** 1–10.
Lewis, C. S. (1961) *A Grief Observed.* London: Faber and Faber (recommended reading).
Parkes, C. M. (1975) *Bereavement: Studies of Grief in Adult Life.* Harmondsworth: Penguin.
Raphael, B. (1984) *The Anatomy of Bereavement: a Handbook for the Caring Professions.* London: Hutchinson (further reading).
Worden, J. W. (1988) *Grief Counselling and Grief Therapy.* London: Tavistock/Routledge.

Further reading

Horn, S. (1989) *Coping with Bereavement: Coming to Terms with a Sense of Loss.* Wellingborough: Thorsons.

Pain

Beales, J. E. (1983) Factors influencing the expectation of pain among patients in a child burns unit. *Burns,* **9,** 187–192.

Egbert I. D. *et al.* (1964) Reduction of post-operative pain by encouragement and instruction of patients, *New Engl. J. Med.,* **270,** 825–827.

Elliott, C. H. and Olson, R. A. (1983) The management of children's distress in response to painful medical treatment for burns injuries, *Behav. Res. Ther.,* **21**(6), 658–683.

Fordyce, W. E. *et al.* (1968) Some implications of learning in problems of chronic pain. *J. Chron. Dis.,* **21,** 179–190.

Katz, E. R. *et al.* (1982a) Self-report and observational measurement of acute pain, fear and behavioural distress in children with leukaemia. Paper presented at the Annual Meeting of the Society of Behavioural Medicine, Chicago.

Katz, E. R. *et al.* (1982b) Behavioural assessment and management of paediatric pain. *Progress in Behaviour Modification,* **18,** 163–193.

Kelley, M. L. *et al.* (1984) Decreasing burned children's pain behaviour. Impacting the trauma of hydrotherapy. *J. Applied Behaviour Analysis,* **17**(2), 147–158.

Melzack, R. (1973) *The Puzzle of Pain.* New York: Basic Books.

Sexual behaviour

Davies, M. (1988) Sexual problems and physical disability. In Goodwill, C. J. and Chamberlain, M. A., eds. *Rehabilitation of the Physically Disabled Adult.* pp. 499–507. London: Croom Helm.

Diamond, M. (1977) Sexuality and the handicapped. In Stubbins, J., ed. *Social and Psychological Aspects of Disability: a Handbook for Practitioners.* Austin, Texas: Pro-Ed.

Grieve, G. P. (1981) *Common Vertebral Joint Problems.* pp. 510–511. Edinburgh: Churchill Livingstone.

Masters, W. H. and Johnson, V. E. (1980) *Human Sexual Inadequacy.* New York: Bantam Books.

Further reading

Davies, M., Hasler, F., Holland, B., Dareborough, A. and Lowden, H. (1982) *Sexuality and the Physically Disabled.* London: SPOD.

Useful addresses

RELATE (National Marriage Guidance Council), Herbert Gray College, Little Church Street, Rugby, Warwickshire CV21 3AP.

SPOD (Sexual and Personal Relationships of the Disabled), 286 Camden Road, London N7 0BJ.

SIA (Spinal Injuries Association), Yeoman House, 76 St James Lanes, London N10 3DF.

Multiple Sclerosis Society, 25 Effie Road, London SW6 1EE.

Spastics Society, 16 Fitzroy Square, London W1P 5HQ.

Part Two

Essential Skills Base

Chapter 6

Working with individuals

Mary Ashwin

The helping relationship

This section will look at the helping relationship from both sides, reviewing the possible reactions of both the service user and the community practitioner and the influences these have on the helping process. First reactions to the practitioners and their interventions are examined after which community practitioners are invited to explore the nature of their own participation in the therapeutic process.

The service user's expectations

It is rare to visit someone who has had no previous contact with helping agencies. If prior contacts have been valued the practitioner will inherit a fund of goodwill. This will lubricate the initial contact while the practitioner clarifies the scope and purpose of the relationship and becomes known and trusted on their own account. If the previous contact has been negative the practitioner may have a more difficult job since these expectations will need to be positively revised if the relationship is to prosper.

Quite apart from previous experiences of helpers, people in pain and distress will often experience some difficulty in involving themselves in new relationships. During a crisis period competent figures may well be related to eagerly, but if the first contact is made during the weary post-crisis phase, little energy may be available for new relationships and the practitioner may be perceived through a prevailing mood of depression.

The practitioner, then, may well be perceived either positively or negatively, not always as a direct result of their own action. It will depend upon the attitudes of the person receiving the service towards other people in general and helpers in particular. Some of the attributes with which practitioners may find themselves endowed, regardless of reality, are:

- *All powerful*
  The practitioner is endowed with the power to solve problems,

cure all ills and produce resources at will. This is an uneasy position, although perhaps initially gratifying, since, eventually, the expectations will be disappointed.

- *Omniscient*
  The practitioner is held in high esteem and looked to for advice and guidance. Again the initial flattery will be quickly overtaken by the realisation that the client is dependent on the practitioner with little capacity to make decisions and act alone.
- *Punitive*
  The practitioner is seen as demanding, difficult to please, who may be treated with respect but will not be trusted with weakness and failings since these would be neither understood nor accepted. The practitioner may well feel some anger and dislike as they are kept out and prevented from establishing a working agreement.
- *Absorbent*
  Here the practitioner is hardly perceived at all except as a sponge which can absorb, in part at least, the torrent of pent-up emotion. The practitioner having afforded such relief, the client will then generate fresh feelings for similar discharge on the next visit. The practitioner may feel overwhelmed, frustrated and incompetent in the face of such a deluge.

The expectations described so far are clearly unhelpful and have to be addressed if progress is to be made.

Other expectations are realistic and appropriate. It is reasonable to expect practitioners to be:

- Competent to practice in their area of specialism.
- Able to communicate effectively with individuals, families and groups.
- Able to liaise effectively with other professionals.
- Operating within a clear ethical framework which will protect the service interests.

Exercise 1

Individually

Review the recent additions to your caseload.

- Have you encountered expectations you felt were unrealistic? If so, what were they?

- How did you set about confirming that you were able to meet legitimate and realistic expectations?

In groups

- Generate a list of expectations which have caused you difficulty in establishing a purposeful relationship.
- Discuss the ways in which users expectations effect the early stages of work.

Barriers to accepting help

A review of the expectations placed upon the helper will show that not all of them are positive, many are ambivalent and some negative. When the fact that some positive expectations are unrealistic and will certainly lead to disillusionment is added, then it is no wonder that it is difficult to establish a good working relationship.

The biblical saying that 'it is more blessed to give than to receive' is one which is often found to be true by the helpers when, through choice or circumstances, they find themselves in the role of the helped. However welcome the help may be, receiving it requires an admission of need which may be painful to acknowledge.

In an ideal situation people will have been referred after consultation and by mutual consent, will be aware of what is being offered and the sort of contribution this will make to the management of their problems. This is often a far cry from the reality of the situation where people may be referred for the sake of others rather than themselves and feel that the whole process of referral by-passes them and adds to their feeling of dis-empowerment.

Both Kennedy (1977) and Egan (1990) make a distinction between resistant and reluctant clients. They do so in contradictory ways, labelling them differently, but observing the same distinction. The distinction is between those for whom the very offer of help is unwelcome and threatening and those who basically want help but who see it as threatening. Egan's distinction will be adopted here.

Resistance

Egan describes resistant people as feeling in some way coerced. This will be expressed as open hostility and rejection, sometimes as a passive refusal to co-operate.

The reasons for resistance are infinitely variable. Some commonly encountered are:

- The help is seen as having no relevance or value.
- There are feelings of being steamrollered by the helping process and being taken over by it.
- Anger that their referral is made to help others rather than for the named person.
- The helper is seen as an unwelcome substitute for another who has rejected them.
- The help is experienced as a confirmation of guilt or a form of punishment for some failing or inadequacy.

Reluctance

This is experienced by those who, although wanting help, have ambivalent feelings about accepting it. This will be experienced by the helper in such ways as feeling dis-empowered, seduced or alienated.

For example:

- An unwillingness to accept the full extent of their neediness, a defence against the magnitude of their problem.
- A need to remain in control of every aspect of life; this is intensified especially when it is reinforced by a growing fear of disintegration.
- Fear of dependency, arising from previous unsatisfactory experiences.
- A desire to maintain the status quo and fear that management of the problem will result in a loss of valued feelings/behaviours/experiences.
- A dread of exposure. Some people have aspects of their lives which seem too bad to be faced, let alone shared. The helper may appear to threaten these defences.
- A fear of rejection. Some people feel that if anyone gets to know them they will reject them because they are neither likeable or lovable.

For both reluctant and resistant people accepting help, however well meant, is a threatening situation. It is important for practitioners to recognise that these barriers have to be approached with respect and cannot be lightly dismissed. Some useful guidelines for working with reluctance and resistance are:

- Seek to understand the reason why work is being resisted.
- Examine your own practice to see if anything in your behaviour may add to the resistance and reluctance you encounter.

- Accept that much of this behaviour is not a direct response to you personally but to you as a helper.
- Remember that defensive behaviour is often unconscious and not therefore deliberately pre-planned by the other person.
- Be open and collaborative in your approach without allowing yourself to be put down or rubbished.
- Find ways of making co-operation attractive and rewarding.
- Know when to quit! People can't be forced into accepting help.

Exercise 2

Individually

Think of a difficult time in your own life when you were at the receiving end of help.

- How did you feel?
- What did you think?
- How did you behave?
- Are there any points you need to remember in your own practice?

In groups

Identify people in your practice for whom accepting help was not easy. Collect together a list of techniques you used in order to establish a working relationship.

Developing trust

The need to see the practitioner as reliable and dependable is an essential prerequisite of effective work. Trust in life is usually established over time, through a body of shared experience, in which the qualities of honesty and sincerity are demonstrated. In most helping contacts professional qualifications and reputation take the place of experience. Most people are capable of sufficient trust to work but some testing out is to be expected.

Fong and Cox (1983) identified six common tests which clients use in a counselling situation. They were:

- *Requesting information*
  These requests were either about the counselling situation or about the counsellors themselves. They seemed to be aimed at

establishing whether the counsellor could understand and accept them.

- *Telling a secret*
  This seemed to be testing how much of themselves it would be safe to disclose without the counsellor appearing to withdraw.
- *Asking a favour*
  This test examined not whether the favour was granted but the way in which it was handled, e.g. the degree of honesty and the reliability of any promises given.
- *Putting oneself down*
  Often this was seen to be an indirect way of asking whether or not the counsellor could accept them.
- *Inconveniencing the counsellor*
  This was seen as testing whether the counsellor was able to set limits and maintain boundaries.
- *Questioning the counsellor's motives*
  Here clients were making sure that the counsellor was not motivated by personal gain, their position largely exploitative. The real question asked was, 'Is your caring real?'

Although formulated in a counselling context these tests occur in any helping relationship. Fong and Cox showed that key areas of concern are acceptance, reliability, boundary keeping and ethical considerations. The practitioner's ability to decode these messages about trust and respond appropriately are valuable skills in relationship building. For some people the ability to experience trust in a helping relationship may be new and valuable, as they experience consistent, non-possessive caring.

Exercise 3

Individually

Reviewing your recent work with people are you able to:

- Identify any of the trust testing strategies outlined above?
- Remember any other incidents where trust has been an issue?

In pairs

Each present an incident where trust was an issue. Focus on:

- How you felt about this test.

- What your response to it was.
- Whether you would still respond in the same way.

The practitioner's contribution to the helping relationship

Because the task of helping people is so complex and the relationships in which it takes place may be far from straightforward, it is important that the practitioner has looked inwards as well as outwards. This introspection should make it easier to determine what the practitioner will contribute to the relationship, what special prejudices, predilections or behaviour will be brought alongside the professional skills on offer. This section seeks to indicate some major areas where the practitioner needs to be self-aware.

Awareness of the influence of the helper's life history

It is not mere chance that some people gravitate to helping roles. The reasons are often complex and contain both conscious and unconscious elements, they include:

- The caring role as a continuation of what happened in the practitioner's family.
- Caring for others as a way of caring for ourselves. Doing to others what we would secretly like done for us.
- Caring for others to make reparation for some failure to care for which the helper feels responsible.
- Caring for others to assert positive caring aspects of the personality and deny aggressive ones.

Some exploration of our motivation to help is important because it often arises from beliefs and feelings which get in the way of good practice. Some such beliefs are:

- I am able to be endlessly available to others.
- My own needs are less important than those of others.
- I am a strong person who can carry others.
- Caring for other people offers me almost total satisfaction.

These are somewhat crudely stated and would never be expressed in these terms but, listening to yourself or colleagues talking about their work, there are some of these beliefs implicit in many conversations. Often these are expressed in relation to taking time off when not feeling well, working unpaid, unwanted overtime, not letting someone else help in a difficult time. Understanding why it is important for us to be carers is the first step towards reducing compulsive and, therefore, irrational elements in our relationship with those who seek help.

Exercise 4

Individually

Examine your own life story and trace the decision to become a professional carer, so far as you are able.

- How do you think your early life history still influences you?
- Can you identify any areas where it has a:
  - positive
  - negative

  influence on your practice?

In pairs

Discuss with a partner (someone from your professional practice) where you felt you failed to achieve all you would have liked in the helping relationship. Try to establish:

1. What made the relationship unsatisfactory for you.
2. How it seemed to be experienced by the other person.
3. What might account for any differences between 1 and 2.

Awareness of the impact of the helper's social and cultural contact

Just as each practitioner has both strengths and needs arising from their particular life experience, so also they will be greatly influenced by the social and cultural background in which they have been brought up. A common observation made by helpers is that they are predominantly white, middle-class women. There are many exceptions to this and the precise truth of it is unimportant. What is more interesting is that it is often expressed as a criticism of the sort of help available. In other words, there is an assumption that help might be more effective if it were offered on the basis of shared experience.

We can do little about the race, sex, class and religion into which we are born. What matters is that as helpers we are aware that our background has provided us with a particular set of assumptions about the world which would, if unchallenged, be taken as universal. These assumptions are further strengthened because we tend to be more comfortable with people who are a bit like us, with whom some things can be taken for granted.

Rejection of our background may only provide us with different types of bias rather than providing greater insight into the lives of others. As helpers, a positive move is to work at understanding the limitations imposed by our cultural heritage as well as acknowledging the many benefits we have derived from it.

Exercise 5

Individually

List the social settings in which you feel comfortable in your private life. Compare this with the settings in which you operate professionally.

- How different are these two lists?
- What enables you to operate effectively as a professional in settings you would find socially difficult?
- What impact may these enabling strategies have on the people with whom you work?

In groups

Discuss how one aspect of your social/cultural background influences your professional work. For example:

- The definition of family and the distribution of family responsibility.
- The importance of education and work.
- Attitudes to money and how it should be used.
- The management of pain and beliefs about it.
- Beliefs about death and the rituals surrounding it.

Awareness of how the helper presents him- or herself to others

Usually it is not a source of mystery to us why some people are constantly experiencing problems with, say, independence. We see the invitation that they offer for interchanges to occur which result in a predictable outcome. Berne (1964) developed a theory of personality and communication in which he describes such interchanges as 'games'. They are one of the ways in which people act out a life script given by others, usually parents, of which they are unaware.

Many helpers are compulsive people watchers and often exhibit great wisdom and insight when they discuss the behaviour and emotions of others. It is a much more slow and painful process becoming aware of ourselves, both in the way we are likely to appear to others and the messages which we send them. It is important for helpers to be as self aware as possible in order to determine the way in which they engage in the helping relationship. Clearly this is especially important when there are difficulties establishing, maintaining or terminating relationships.

Johari's window (Figure 6.1) is a useful illustration of self-awareness in communication. (It is so called after its two originators, Joseph Luft and Harrington Ingham 1979.) They see areas of awareness like four sections of a window. They consist of:

- The part known only to ourselves.
- The part known only to others.
- The part known to ourselves and others.
- The part known by neither ourselves or others.

They suggest that for communication to become more effective we have to work at the areas of which we are, as yet, unaware. This

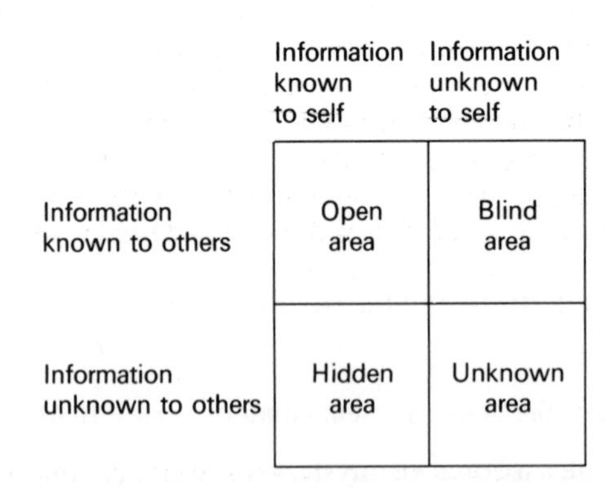

Figure 6.1 The Johari window: areas of awareness

is because we can only effectively use those parts of ourselves of which we are fully conscious.

We will look in the next section at self-awareness and concentrate here on ourselves in relation to others (this is a difficult distinction to make so both sections must really be seen as part of a whole). This having been said, there are things we can do to become more aware of the way in which we present ourselves to others. They include:

- Asking friends or colleagues for their first impression of us and how accurate they now feel this to be.
- Watching for any patterns that emerge in our practice, recurring situations, similar communication sequences.
- Listen to feedback from all sources, the service consumer (patients, clients etc), colleagues, managers, other professionals.
  - Is there a consistent message?
  - What are the differences between the messages?
  - Is there consistency of feedback from particular sources? For example, do I consistently get good feedback from service users and poor feedback from managers? If so, why might this be?
- Identify any differences in the feedback received about ourselves in personal, intimate roles with that in professional roles.
- Is there a marked difference in the feedback that we receive in one to one situations to that which we receive in group settings?

All this sounds rather simple and perhaps rather too intense. In fact it requires considerable openness which is often uncomfortable and sometimes painful. It is because of the risky nature of this enterprise that so many people remain comparatively unaware of their social impact. Without this knowledge, however, no matter how perceptive we are about the observed behaviour of others, we may often fail to understand what has provoked it because we will have excluded the impact of our own behaviour.

Often quite simple adjustments to our social presentations can improve the quality of all interactions, smiling more or less frequently, or talking in a rather more or less decisive way.

Exercise 6

Individually

Identify whether there is any consistent feedback about which you are unhappy. In order for it to be changed, what adjustments should be made in the environment or in yourself? If in yourself:

- How?
- When?

In pairs

Discuss the exercise above, taking it in turns to discuss any problems you may have identified. Test out the extent to which your perceptions of yourself are shared by your partner.

Awareness of the helper's inner life

Helpers are professionally equipped with certain knowledge and skills which place them in a special relationship with those whom they help. It is a powerful position which will be reviewed again in the section on ethics. Personally, however, they are as prone to difficulty as anyone else. Some feel that the very need to be in a helping profession indicates a certain vulnerability as well as a certain strength. Because helpers meet people when they are in special need it is very important that they are in touch with their own feelings.

Some people might argue that if the contact is professional then personal feelings should be kept firmly in check. There is a very real sense in which this is true; most helpers at one time or another have become over-involved with the people with whom they work and experienced the problems that this can cause. The best helpers, however, do make something of themselves available and it is this 'non-possessive warmth' described by Rogers (1961) which gives life to the relationships and supports the other person while they work.

It is the need to offer emotional as well as clinical support which makes case-loads demanding. The ability to be available to people in this way, without becoming bogged down in a morass of feeling, is achieved through the helper being aware of the feelings which this person provokes without letting it impinge negatively on their relationship. The times when helpers are in the most danger is when they sail blithely into situations and realise too late what has been going on. Awareness does not mean morbid self-obsession; it means recognising feeling and dealing with it appropriately and professionally.

There are a number of ways in which you could improve your understanding of yourself. All of these take time and some will not appeal or be useful to you. The following list is offered to spark off your own ideas of how to develop a better understanding of yourself amid the demands of a busy professional life.

- Read again some of the books on social, developmental, cognitive and behavioural psychology which you probably studied as part of your training. This time read them specifically with yourself in mind.

  Transactional analysis (TA) was mentioned earlier. Founded by Berne, it is a useful tool for this sort of work. Ellis founded yet another therapy, rational emotive therapy (RET) and also offers an interesting way of analysing how thinking influences behaviour. He discusses two types of self-appraisal: rational and irrational, offering a useful checklist of irrational beliefs. Many helpers suffer, for instance, from the irrational belief that 'I should be thoroughly competent, adequate and achieving in all things I do and be recognised as such.'
- Devise a list of your strengths and needs, noticing the relationship between them. The aspects of ourselves which are strong will often have corresponding weaknesses. Flexibility can deteriorate into disorganisation, courage into rashness and warmth into over-involvement. Make plans for how your needs might be met.
- Keep a journal in which you explore: (i) your current activities, (ii) your thoughts and (iii) your feelings. It will be very informative which of these three aspects of your life is more readily explored.
- Review your current support system – is it adequate? If formal support is rather scanty, have you a good informal support network? Sometimes this can be exploited more effectively by coming to an agreement, with a colleague, to devote an equal amount of time each to listening to and supporting each other at the same recognised time during the working month.
- If you feel that there are unresolved problems in your personal life which interfere with your professional development, it could be very worthwhile doing some work with another professional helper such as a counsellor.

The practitioner's attitude to helping

A study of our motivations to become helpers and an appraisal of our strengths and needs will probably destroy the delusion that the helper is somehow different and special and the person in need is particularly weak and inadequate. There are times when we all need help in order to develop healthy coping strategies and we may do this through family and friends or with the help of other professional people. Egan (1990) pinpoints two crucial attitudes and stresses the need that they should find expression in the way helpers relate and work with those they meet.

Genuinness

Egan describes genuine people as 'those who are at home with themselves'. (He was talking, at the time, to those who wanted to be counsellors, but it applies equally to all helpers.) Being genuine assures that the helpers are not hiding behind a glossy professional facade, or feeling that they are able to know everything and remain permanently calm, unruffled and responsive. In other words, they are able to accept their own fallibility and its consequences.

Genuine helpers will, therefore be those who are:

- Open in communication, avoiding games and hidden agendas.
- Able to behave assertively and consistently without defensiveness.
- Able to make available their therapeutic skills without retreating behind a defensive professionalism.
- Able to respond spontaneously to each person and situation as it arises.

Being genuine is not easy; everyone from time to time escapes into some well-worn patter or shrinks behind their protective uniform. Such strategies are perhaps inevitable in a stressful working environment. It is important, though, for the helper to realise they are about professional survival as well as professional identity. If overused these techniques may come to act as a barrier between yourself and the other person, so that no real encounter ever occurs. If this happens a vital ingredient of the helping relationship will be lost.

Exercise 7

Individually or in groups

Review your last week of practice. Identify any instances where you put up the emotional shutters and retreated behind a 'professional' facade.

- What were the circumstances which led to this action?
- With whom were you involved?
- What does this tell you about your professional practice?
- What does it tell you about yourself?

Respect

Another essential attitude is that helpers should respect those with whom they work. We are all very sensitive to the degree of respect we receive, even if we don't talk about it, or even think about it in those terms. People often emerge from some professional encounters muttering darkly about having been treated like an idiot or having been made to feel really bad. This isn't always the helper's fault, as we discussed earlier, but unless people feel valued they are unlikely to be very trusting or cooperative.

This does not mean that helpers have to become hopelessly idealistic about everyone they treat. Being respectful means that the helper believes that, just as everyone is fallible and vulnerable, so too everyone has an inherent value. It is the recognition that people have the ability to make choices, both positive and negative, that it is possible to review these choices and make changes in their lives. Those who work with people who are dying often report how positive change is possible among all the negative change associated with death.

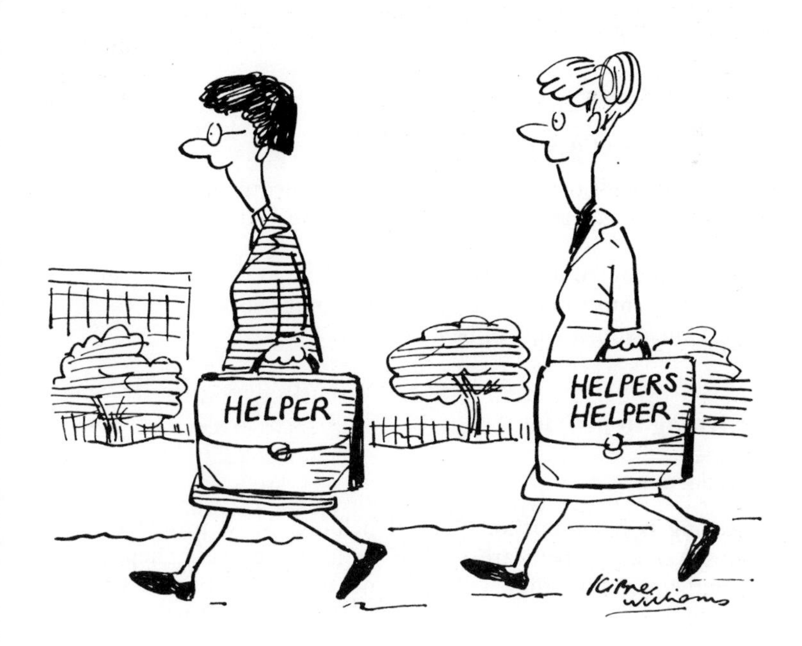

Respect for others is a source of hope and encouragement and a loss of respect is one of the causes of practitioner burn-out. Like being genuine, being respectful, at times, can require work on our part. This is particularly true when the helper is working with those who are reluctant and resistant or where, realistically, the potential for change is limited.

Most practitioners would protest that openness and respect are basic to their practice, but this is not always apparent to those with whom they work. There are very simple ways of demonstrating respect and when such signs are absent service users will often feel put down or neglected, even if no such thing was intended.

Ways of showing respect

- Being on time for appointments.
- Addressing the person by name.
- Avoiding interruptions.
- Valuing positive aspects of the service user.
- Seeking to understand the problem from their stand point.
- Respecting other people's opinions when they are different from your own.
- Showing we value people's capacity to make choices and act upon them.
- Supporting someone in the coping strategy of their choice.

Exercise 8

Individually or in groups

Looking realistically at your working schedule, are there any ways you could avoid any of the following, if they occur:

- Being late or unreliable.
- Being interrupted when you are helping people.
- Conveying a sense of being rushed.

Listening to people

Introduction

Listening is an important part of helping. Most people who see themselves as helpers are careful to listen to their clients. In a strengths/needs list they will often mention listening as a strength. Despite this, however, it is quite likely that not all those with whom they work will feel as if they have really been heard. This failure of communication occurs when, for example,

- People feel the social distance is too great between themselves and the helper.
- Helpers fail to convey effectively their feelings of concern.
- People have come to believe no one listens to them.
- Helpers appear hurried, pre-occupied and under pressure.

The list could continue because effective two-way communication is not easy to achieve at the best of times and when people are burdened, physically, mentally or emotionally, they need someone who is able to facilitate the process for them. The demonstration of respect and genuinness has an important contribution to make but helpers need to develop their communication skills so that these attitudes are obvious and unmistakable.

Communication consists of both messages that use words and those which do not; in other words, verbal and non-verbal transactions. This section on listening will focus largely on the non-verbal communication of the helper, although of course all this equally applies to those with whom we are working. It will include suggestions on how to listen with greater understanding and describes the sort of conditions that are likely to hinder effective communication and those which will enhance it.

Components of non-verbal communication

Non-verbal communication includes all the ways in which we communicate other than the actual words we use. Since they occur while the other person is talking they are an essential part of listening. Talkers frequently scan the listener for such signs as withdrawal, flagging or heightened interest or hostility.

Exercise 9

Individually or in groups

List as many of the non-verbal signals which take place within a professional encounter as possible (e.g. facial expression and posture).

The list you generate will incude all, or many, of the following:

Proximity and space. This may vary throughout an average session, depending upon your professional tasks. In many medical settings the usual rules about how close we get to each other are often overturned because of the nature of the work. This is compensated for by other distancing devices such as wearing uniforms which emphasise the professional nature rather that the personal nature of the interaction.

One of the ways in which we demonstrate an awareness of the nature of a relationship, especially such aspects as dominance and intimacy, is through social positioning. The person who is perceived as being the most powerful dictates the positions adopted. In general this will be the helper, providing yet another insight into the vulnerability of those we help.

An awareness of our power in this area should alert us to the need to manage it with sensitivity. Helpers should be assertive enough to create the right forum for listening, where the faces of both people are clearly visible without undue strain. This is not always that easy when people are sitting or lying in positions which do not correspond well to either normal standing or sitting positions.

When both are seated, it is important that the space is small enough to allow the person to speak freely and yet distant enough to prevent the feeling of being crowded and of privacy being invaded. Research shows that there is rough agreement about the right space for private conversation, referred to as the 'intimate zone', but it is not universal. Every so often there will be people who deviate from the usual expectations, which can result in discomfort for both.

Gaze. As in the case of proximity, needs vary. Some people prefer more eye-contact than others and personal needs will change according to the situation. Like proximity it is connected with intimacy and privacy. Lovers gaze into each other's eyes, while, in a crowded train, eye-contact is avoided to counteract the enforced proximity.

Very often some negotiations take place until this feels right. People may indicate they feel uncomfortable by avoiding eye-contact, by looking away or shielding their face with their hands. In most cultures a fixed stare is seen as a challenge, so that when looking at another's face gaze is usually centred around the region of the mouth.

People often talk best when they feel attended to but relatively unobserved and when the attention of the other person is to some extent occupied elsewhere. Hairdressers often receive very intimate confidences. This seems to be something to do with the intimacy created by the touching combined with the safety of their preoccupation with the hair. A similar situation arises for many helpers whose role involves both touch and proximity and where eye-contact may be less frequent because of the activities in which they are involved.

Posture. The helper is often engaged in some task which involves them being in a very different position from that which normally would be chosen if listening were their only occupation. The back of someone who is listening, however, does look different from someone who is tense and preoccupied.

When sitting talking, a relaxed and open posture is the most likely one to encourage communication. Here the word open, as in relationships, means avoiding any gestures which may look defensive. Folded arms create an impression that someone is protecting themselves. Some people feel crossed legs create a similar impression but this tends to be such a common sitting position that this objection seems, somehow, rather less convincing.

It can be helpful to check your posture from time to time. Most people have had the experience of catching themselves unaware in a shop window and being quite surprised at what they see. Tension creeps up during a rather fraught day and whitened knuckles may give an emotional state away before we have properly registered it.

Touch. Many community practitioners frequently touch their clients as part of their everyday work. Because we live in a society where we touch infrequently outside the family or in sexual contacts, this is something which has to be re-coded as a professional rather than a personal activity. This is usually achieved by formalities and routines which safeguard those involved. The widespread use of uniforms in medical settings is an example of this.

Usually in community-based practice there is rather less formality and routine so, occasionally, the situation can result in misunderstandings. People starved of friendly warmth can become hungry for physical contact and relish it, even if they know that it is offered as part of a treatment plan. Sometimes, of course, the practitioner will be using touch as an expression of their feelings at a particular time. Holding someone's hand can be more powerfully comforting than words.

Touching is also demonstrative of power, putting your arm around someone may be a gesture of concern, but it can also be received as a signal of dominance. People may resent such gestures, seeing them as patronising. For example, women often comment that men are far more likely to put their arm around a woman than the other way round. This may well be something to do with height, but height also conveys dominance.

The problem of relying too heavily on touch as a way of communicating is that it is as open to misinterpretation as any other method and is very powerful. As already indicated, the areas of confusion are likely to be around dominance or sexuality. If misunderstandings do occur, it is important that helpers are comfortable enough to raise the issue and discuss it.

A useful question to ask when gratuitously touching someone (i.e. not as part of a treatment) is 'Why am I touching this person; is it for myself or for them?' It is also important to be similarly questioning of the person who seeks contact with the helper. Gut reactions about the safety of situations may be reliable but are not always so. Practitioners need to be clear about their own boundaries, assertive in their defence and able to articulate their reasons for defending them.

Exercise 10

Individually

Consider the following:

- How often are you in physical contact with people in your community?
- Is there any qualitative difference between some contacts and others? (e.g. are factors like age and sex significant?)
- What are your own personal rules about the use of touch?
- Has touch ever been an issue for you in your work?

In groups

Discuss the way in which you use touch outside specific treatments.

- Are there any significant variations within the group?
- What advice would you want to offer a new community practitioner?

Vocal behaviour. Vocal behaviour includes everything to do with the way we speak apart from the actual words we say. The tone in which something is said is often felt by the listener to be more important than the actual words. 'It is not what you said but the tone in which you said it.' Understanding will be similarly modified by speed, emphasis, pitch, pauses and assertiveness.

People often experience discontent with their helpers because of the way in which things are said. 'She said I was to ask if I had any questions, but I could tell she was in a hurry so I didn't like to.' 'He seemed very cool and off-hand and I didn't feel he was at all interested.' People in the less dominant role usually watch the behaviour of the dominant person carefully, as they feel they have more to lose.

It is very important not to take basic things for granted such as:

Understanding. Things which are everyday and ordinary to one person are new and confusing to another. Familiarity may desensitise us to this. This has important implications for the speed with which we talk, the length of the words we use and the complexity of the sentences in which we express ourselves. It can be equally damaging to assume there is a problem with comprehension because someone is of a different race, age or social group. Checking out understanding in the early stages of a contact and sensitive observation should avoid such problems.

Audibility. The conditions in which a community practitioner operates can make audibility a problem. People often keep a television on permanently for company and do not immediately think of turning it off unless you ask them if they will. Other people may be engaged in noisy activities nearby. Sometimes the nature of the task means that communication does not take place face to face, so many visual clues are lost. People are often reluctant to admit to having difficulties so, as in the case of understanding, it is important to check whether or not you can be heard clearly, particularly if you know that your voice presents people with problems.

Personal style. The way in which people speak is, in this culture, one of the ways in which people are assigned to certain social and regional groups. Similarity is reassuring, differences will be noted and can increase the feeling of social distance. The way in which language is used varies considerably, as does the choice of words themselves. These differences will influence the understanding and the audibility of what we say and as practitioners we need to be aware of our own peculiarities and make allowances for them.

Exercise 11

In pairs

Make a video tape in which each partner has 5 minutes to explore some problem.

Replay the video and discuss with your partner:

- Characteristics of your verbal style (tone, speed etc.).
- Your use of language.
- How enabled your partner felt by you when you were in the listening role.

Note. The use of video may be uncomfortable if you are not used to it but it does provide very good learning material. If anything it has a rather flattening effect so that emotions may not come over as clearly as they do in real life.

In groups

Discuss the making of the video. Examine:

- Your reactions to the experience.
- What you have learnt about yourself as a result of the exercise.

Facial expression. Because we are conscious that facial expressions can betray our feelings, most people become rather skilled at masking emotions which they wish to conceal. It is easy to misinterpret facial expressions even when people are not carefully controlling them. Despite the fact that we know it is an unreliable source of information, we frequently scan the faces of those with whom we talk for information. Mouths and eyebrows are particularly mobile and determine facial expression to a large degree.

As helpers it is important to give out messages which are clear and facilitate our task. If we are somewhat solemn faced it is important to remember to smile to reassure someone who is feeling nervous. It is always important to remember that our facial expression supports what we are saying. It is confusing if we are raising a very serious issue with a laugh that belies its importance. We are guilty from time to time of giving double messages and offering ourselves escape routes at the expense of directness and honesty. Such behaviour ultimately undermines the helping relationship as many people may begin to doubt how genuine we are.

Exercise 12

In pairs

Using the video tape made for the previous exercise, play each 5 minutes through without sound. Decide:

- Whether your face is expressing the emotions you remember feeling at the time.
- Whether your partner is able to interpret your feelings correctly.

Physical presence. There is something very distinct about each of us. We have a certain shape, smell and appearance. Some aspects of this we are more aware of than others. We usually have to think to some extent about what we wear because of the effort of getting dressed, although the impact this has on others may be less obvious to us. People who feel themselves, in some way, to be markedly different from those around them, will be more self-conscious than others.

It is important for helpers to be aware of this overall self presentation and hopefully the work in the previous exercises will have heightened your awareness. There may well be some aspects in your self presentation which operate quite powerfully, especially in first meetings. Knowledge of them may allow you to off-set aspects which could appear off-putting or intimidating to others.

Exercise 13

Individually

Identify someone with whom you have worked whose presentation caused you difficulties.

- Were these difficulties eventually resolved?
- If so, how did this happen?
- What can you learn from this experience in relation to your own practice?

Listening and observation

Just as it is important that we become more aware of the non-verbal messages we are sending, so it is of equal importance to carefully observe those we receive. Listed earlier were all those signals which were under the helper's control; our observations should also include all those responses like trembling, blushing, sweating and quickened breathing which occur in stressful situations.

Non-verbal communication is generally regarded as a valuable source of information because it is thought to be less easily disguised and manipulated than speech, but the real problem for the helper is interpreting what you have observed. For example, if you commonly blush with embarrassment, it is easy to assume that everyone does the same, but there are many other causes of blushing.

The only way of accurately interpreting these signals is to observe them over a period paying special attention to the social context in which they occur. Very often the helper has to act and respond without such information so it is necessary for some acknowledgement of our comparative ignorance. 'You seem to be embarrassed by that', for example, offers the other person the opportunity of saying, 'Oh no, I was just rather excited about it.' A categorical 'You are embarrassed, there is really no need to be', might leave the person feeling misunderstood and irritated.

Two useful measures to bear in mind when observing non-verbal behaviour are:

1. *The level of congruence.* How well the verbal and non-verbal messages seem to fit. Is 'I am really glad about that' supported by all the usual non-verbal behaviour associated with pleasure? If they do seem in general agreement, is the level of feeling equal in both sets of messages?
2. *The degree of confusion.* In some ways the opposite side of the coin from 1. For example, someone tells a story which would seem to be very sad in a rather humorous way. This may leave us very undecided as to the way in which they really feel. Pointing out your confusion is often the best way of solving the mystery. 'You make it sound very funny, but it sounds a pretty awful situation to me. I wonder how you really feel.' This gives people permission to express any feelings they like; colluding with the laughter might reinforce their own prohibition on grief. It is important then to note the confusion and, whenever possible, resolve it.

Exercise 14

Individually

Think of a situation in your practice where you feel, in

retrospect, you misinterpreted what you were being told. Could the misunderstanding be attributed to:

- The other person's difficulty in expressing themselves?
- Your lack of knowledge of this person's behaviour?
- Any special pressures in the situation which inhibited your receptiveness?

What could you do to try to avoid such misunderstandings in future?

Barriers to listening

As the last exercise may have illustrated for you, listening well makes great demands on the helper, observing carefully both what occurs and the situation in which it occurs. With such a wealth of information we are bound to be selective in our observations and so much will be lost. Helpers have to minimise the dangers arising from our failures to observe or rightly interpret the situation. Things to avoid include:

- Having such a fixed view of the person and/or situation that evidence that does not fit is filtered out.
- Preoccupation with matter which has priority for us rather than the person with whom we are working.
- Accepting what is said at face value and not allowing for defensive behaviour, e.g. worry expressed as anger or misery as opting-out.
- Ignorance of other people's culture, e.g. the different meanings given to illness and acceptable ways of expressing discomfort.
- Running away from issues which we find painful. Every now and then a helper is caught on a raw spot and the immediate response is to get away from the pain. Staying with the other person and our own pain is not easy.

Exercise 15

In groups

Discuss any difficulties you experience in listening attentively in your practice.

- Check out the severity of these problems and the regularity with which they occur.
- How far do you see yourself able to limit the problems and improve your listening skills?

Listening and understanding

We have already looked at the problems of making sense of non-verbal messages. As might be expected, understanding what we hear is no easier. Kennedy (1977) offers a framework for listening which makes us alive to the various facets of what we are told in a way which enriches our understanding.

He alerts us to five components of any story which we are told. These are:

1. *The feeling tone.* No matter what the content of the story, e.g. difficulties in dressing or a disagreement with a relative, what is the predominant feeling throughout? Listen for the emotion which colours each twist of the story, e.g. anger, despair, determination.
2. *The perspective.* Here Kennedy advises listening to the way in which time is viewed. Is the emphasis on the past or is the future important? Is someone still preoccupied with mourning a lost way of life or are they able to make future plans based on present reality?
3. *Prospects.* The listener's concern here is with how challenge and difficulty are viewed by the speaker. How do they rate themselves in a tight corner? Are they hopeful or despairing?
4. *Central identification.* How does the person talk about themselves? Is it as someone who does things or as someone to whom things happen? Are they active or passive in their experience of life? Are they taking responsibility for themselves or blaming other people?
5. *The theme.* Listening for themes involves identifying the common thread which runs through all the various stories someone tells us. Without being fully aware of it, people select stories which illustrate their central preoccupation. It may be stories which are full of conflict or ones in which the person feels that those around have failed to be properly supportive. The possibilities are numerous. Skilful listeners will not just listen to the details of the story but be asking why this particular story has been chosen and how it relates to others that have been told. Kennedy suggests that when stories are repeated it is because counsellors have failed to understand and respond appropriately.

Most professional practitioners will have met people where one or other of these five components have been particularly pronounced so this kind of analysis will not be new. Thinking about communication in this very focused way may speed up and improve understanding.

Egan (1990) offers similar advice to listeners. He emphasises, however, the need for helpers to encourage people to be specific in three particular areas.

1. *Feelings.* The topic is clear even though the feelings may be confused.
2. *Experiences.* All the things which happen to a person from being run over by a bus to being told to sit still as a child.
3. *Behaviours.* All the things which are done by someone; running, sleeping, thinking, day dreaming.

Like Kennedy, he makes the point that people who talk mainly in terms of experience are often rather passive, whilst people who talk in terms of behaviour tend to be active and accepting of responsibility for their part in whatever is going on. If people are to involve themselves in actions to manage their problems the helper will notice that movement is required from the passive to the active voice.

It is also useful to note how much feeling is expressed and named or how much is just implied. Some people find the direct expression of feeling very threatening and this can create misunderstandings. The feelings that seem reasonable to us in a particular circumstance may be different from those actually experienced.

This thoughtful, analytical listening is very demanding and probably cannot be achieved all the time. What is important is that the helper is capable of focusing on the story, in this very detailed way, when this is appropriate, to ensure that useful work can begin or continue.

Structured listening

Most helpers have had the uncomfortable experience of knowing they have run out of time with someone who shows no sign of willingly letting go. All the way to the door and down the path the outpourings continue and it feels that if one looked back along the street they would still be there desperately trying to catch your attention.

Such situations can produce a number of emotions in the practitioner; anger at the unreasonable level of demand, guilt that it can not be satisfied, sadness because of the desperation which provoked it. These emotions in turn can be expressed by avoidance, by placating or by compensating them on the next visit. All of these actions confirm the special nature of the person's difficulty and may be seen as, in some ways, lacking in respect.

If we believe that people are able to change their behaviour and are responsible for their lives, there is no need to give them special time which will be taken from someone else who is more co-operative but, perhaps, not less needy. What we should be offering is a full and competent service. The helper's responsibility is to spell out what this service will entail so that realistic expectations can be established.

The desperation described in the doorstep drama is born of the belief that no one is able to tolerate them or listen to them. Our hasty retreat down the garden path confirms this feeling. The firm structure and boundaries suggested may at first be resisted and resented, but this will eventually be outweighed by the fact that, unlike others, we return.

Community practice tends to be hectic and some of the guilt mentioned earlier may be based on the fact that visits have to be rushed and the time available for a particular person may vary. All the practitioner can do in this situation is to state assertively what the boundaries are for a particular day. It is not easy; so many people are very lonely and sad and may have no one else to call for that day. All we can offer is a good, caring service, delivered with respect.

Exercise 16

In pairs

With a partner review a recent interview where boundaries were a problem. Analyse the experience in terms of:

- What was expected of the worker.
- The time available for the interview.
- Your feelings about the relationship between 1 and 2.
- Your ability to observe the time boundaries.
- Your ability to maintain a good working relationship.

In groups

Share the main difficulties which helpers identified in their interviews. Devise a list of possible strategies which might address the problems.

Talking to people

Introduction

The quality of the helping relationship will be influenced not only by how well we are able to listen and make sense of what we hear but also how we respond and communicate that understanding. There are a number of communication skills which can be used in order to make the best use of the time available for work with any particular person or group. They are:

- demonstrating our understanding by using *empathy*,
- eliciting information and guiding interviews by using various types of *questioning*,
- encouraging and facilitating change by various types of *challenge*.

All of these techniques, whether you describe them in this way or not, will already be part of your professional style of communicating, just as we all use them in everyday speech. What this section hopes to encourage is the recognition of them as specific types of verbal intervention, each of which has particular uses. This is important since all of them can be used more or less appropriately, either facilitating or hindering the process of change.

Some helpers find this analysis of their conversations rather upsetting. They say that it robs them of their spontaneity and they become less effective. In the short term becoming self-conscious in this way is inhibiting and just getting on with it may seem preferable. In the long term helpers who take the trouble to improve their communication skills find that this is of use to them in every area of their lives. Relationships thrive or wither largely as a result of the quality of communication that is achieved within them. The prized spontaneity is not permanently lost but returns as the skills become firmly integrated into the professional repertoire.

In the following sections the skills will be described and checklists offered as a guide to their appropriate usage, forming a brief overview of key techniques.

Empathy

1. What it is

'Empathy' is now used in a very general way to include anything which aspires to being sensitive and responsive to individual needs.

Carl Rogers (1961) developed a counselling style which relied heavily on the use of empathy. He described it as 'entering into the perceptual world of the other and becoming thoroughly at home in it'. It is described in everyday language as putting yourself in someone else's shoes or seeing the world from another's point of view. When used to describe a communication skill it means not only achieving this understanding but being able to convey that understanding to the person concerned.

The basis of empathy is reflection. Reflection consists of listening for the central message which is being expressed and then repeating it back in your own words. Empathy is one step further on because here the helper reflects back both the *content* of what is said and the *feeling* that accompanies it. This feeling may have been expressed verbally or non-verbally. Given the earlier discussion of the difficulties in interpreting both non-verbal and verbal messages, it is clearly not that easy.

Example

Jackie, the mother of a 3½-year-old boy, collapses into a chair.

Jackie. Paul has been an absolute pain at playgroup again today. When I went to collect him the supervisor told me he'd taken over a toy car they all like and tried to stop anyone else playing with it. He really doesn't seem to like it there very much since Mrs Parry left but I feel it's important for him to get used to being with other children before he goes to school.

Helper. It seems as if Paul's behaviour at playgroup has really started to worry you.

Jackie. Yes, he is fine as long as he is the centre of attention but . . .

This very straightforward reflection encouraged Jackie to continue talking about her worries in more detail.

Exercise 17

In groups

Sit in a circle. Someone begins by telling their neighbour on the left a brief account of some event or concern. 'My journey to work today' provides a useful starter. It may be useful to use the formula 'so you feel . . . because . . .', for the neighbour to reflect on what they see as the main emotional and factual gist of the story. The narrator confirms that this is an accurate reflection before the reflector turns to talk to the person on their left.

Example

Narrator. Well, it was pouring with rain and the traffic was really awful. I just crawled along all the way and when I got to the car park it was full again. Altogether it wasn't a good start.

Reflector. So you feel rather deflated because you had such a stressful journey today.

In pairs

Each person has 5 minutes to talk about some current concern which they feel able to share. The listener tries, at least once, to reflect both the content and the feeling of what is being expressed. Make sure that the feeling is named. It's easy to say 'you feel' without doing so. For example:

'You feel you've got a lot to do', instead of
'You feel *anxious* because you've got a lot to do.'

2. *How to use empathy*

Empathy may seem obvious and easy but it requires considerable practice to use it effectively, as you may have already found in the preceding exercises. Perhaps, as you took the role of the person being listened to, you also experienced how good it was when you had been clearly understood. Some points to bear in mind when you are using empathic responding are:

- Keep your responses fairly brief; they should focus rather than confuse.
- Try to identify what is central and reflect on that.
- Try to match the intensity of feeling contained in your reflections to that expressed e.g. do not say 'furious' when the other person has said 'a bit cross'.
- Use with reasonable frequency. It is important to check that your understanding is correct, especially if the material is complex.

- Make contradiction possible by not sounding too dogmatic, i.e. use words like 'perhaps' or 'it seems as if'.
- Be assertive, ask for space if the speaker does not offer it. For example, 'Could I just make sure I've understood you correctly'. Follow this with an empathic response.
- Base your empathic response on the full range of communication, not just the words used, e.g. facial expression, body language or the way in which it was said.

3. Why empathy is important

Helpers are very privileged when they are allowed into the lives of those with whom they work. They often experience good feelings because they feel trusted and respected. It is important that the service user's loss of privacy is rewarded by evidence of respect and understanding. Empathy is a valuable tool in conveying these messages. Its use can enable someone to:

- Feel accepted and heard by the helper.
- Review what they have been saying.
- Arrive at a clearer understanding of their situation.
- Correct any misunderstanding the helper may have.

Helpers use empathy in order to:

- Show they have real concern and are therefore attending carefully.
- Test that they have interpreted messages correctly.
- Stay focused on the needs of the service user.
- Encourage exploration of those areas which will illuminate the problem.

4. Cautions about the use of empathy

- Empathy, like every other technique, has to be used sensitively. There are times when silence or some non-verbal gesture will seem more appropriate.
- If the formula approach, 'You feel . . . because . . .' is used too frequently it can become obvious and rather irritating.
- People who are rather frightened of feelings may find the clear labelling of them involved in empathy very threatening.

To conclude, empathy is a useful technique which demonstrates the helper's willingness to listen to the other person, and try to understand their problems. Its use helps practitioners to avoid sounding judgemental, rushing into giving advice or leaping into premature problem solving before the problem has been fully explored.

Exercise 18

Either: in groups of three

Interview as before but this time use an observer. Work for 10 minutes in each role (helper/service user/observer). After each interview the observer will offer feedback on the helper's use of empathy.

Or: in pairs

Working in pairs, interview as before, but this time using an audio or video recorder. After each of you has been interviewed play them back. Note both the quantity and quality of your empathic responses.

Questions

1. The different types of question

Unlike empathy, everybody knows what questions are. They are a vitally important learning strategy. People who have looked after little children will have felt positively assaulted, at times, by an endless stream of 'why' questions as children try to make sense of the world around them. Similarly, the community practitioner, beginning work with someone new, will have a list of things they need to know in order to find the best way of helping. Hopefully they will also allow space for the other person to ask questions of them.

Questions in everyday practice are therefore a device by which we obtain necessary information within the helping relationship. They are often based on a different perception of the world from that of the person being questioned, derived from a body of specialised knowledge of which the general public are largely ignorant. Questions are a way of the helper intervening, controlling and directing the communication.

There are a number of different ways of posing questions which vary in the measure of control they seek to place upon the respondent. They include the following:

Leading questions. These are perhaps the most closed type of question of all. Closed, in this context, means the measure of constraint or limitation exerted by the questioner. Leading questions do, if answered, commit the respondent to a position which they may well not wish to hold. 'When did you stop beating your wife?' is the old chestnut often used to illustrate this. As practitioners, we like to think we avoid them because the answers tend to be unreliable. I suspect we are all guilty of them from time to time, e.g. 'Which of these two treatments has helped you most?' (the assumption being that both have been helpful).

Closed questions. This type of question is useful if specific information is required; 'What is your name?' Unlike leading questions, they do not commit the person to a particular position but they do limit the response to a particular area. They may vary in the degree to which they are closed. 'Which of these do you prefer?' offers limited choice but still focuses the discussion quite clearly. A simple test of whether questions are closed or open (the reverse) is to see if you can answer them with a yes or no. 'Is it rather too hot for you?'; 'Am I speaking loudly enough?'.

They are valuable time savers and often help set a mood of co-operation and purposeful activity. They are less good if you want to develop a topic in a way which will tell you something about someone's priorities or opinions.

Open questions. An open question leaves respondents free to explore it in any way they please. It will often begin with words such as What, Why or How. These are often quite difficult questions to answer and someone subjected to a battery of them may well feel under verbal attack.

Some people fall into the trap of asking a good open question and then closing it by suggesting answers if there is a slight pause. People need time to think and if the silence is uncomfortable fill it with something neutral like 'It's a difficult question, don't hurry.' If you don't wait you will never know whether they really agree with your suggestion or whether they just found it easier to go along with the professional.

Statements which invite elaboration. Because questions do constitute a verbal demand it helps to avoid their over use. One strategy is to show that you need more information because of your confusion/ ignorance etc. without actually asking for it directly. These statements of the practitioner's need may include such phrases as;

'I'm not quite sure how you felt about your parents' divorce.'

or 'Sometimes it is difficult to know what you mean when you talk about laziness.'
or 'I'm puzzled by what this means to you.'

They are somewhat less overt in their demands and so can be brushed aside or the respondent may simply agree they are not simple issues. The questioner probably will have marked them down as issues which could be usefully explored, however, so they may well not have been wasted.

Other techniques which are used include that of emphasising a particular word which has been used and repeating it as a question:

'I feel that no one in my family cares about me at all.'
'No one?'
'Well, perhaps my daughter.'

Again this can be seen less threatening as it is based on something someone has said themselves rather than coming entirely from the helper.

There are also a number of non-specific verbal and non-verbal promptings which include all the grunts, hmmms and head-nods which are commonly used to encourage people to say more. They obviously are not really questions at all but they serve a similar purpose, in the sense that they are encouragement for someone to go on and say more.

Exercise 19

Individually or in groups

Try to generate at least one example of each of the following:

- A leading question.
- A statement which invites elaboration.
- An open question.

2. *How to use questions*

The danger of someone feeling threatened by the over-use of questions has already been mentioned. Putting people on the spot may have value in certain circumstances but generally it does not help engender feelings of trust and confidence. Too intrusive questions may provoke responses like 'Why do you want to know?', 'What business is it of yours?', 'Who are you going to tell?' even if they are not openly voiced.

Some guidelines are:

- Use open questions or questioning statements if you want to encourage further exploration.
- If you have just asked an explorative question (as opposed to a straightforward closed one) and received an answer, respond with empathy before moving on to another one. It can seem sometimes as if helpers are insatiable and ungrateful in their demands for yet more.
- Do not get carried away by your own need to know. Always consider whether the answer to a question will help in the understanding and managing of presenting problems.
- Be sensitive in your use of questions: the more pertinent they are, the more likely it is that answering them will be difficult and perhaps painful.
- Be willing to accept areas of uncertainty; there are some things people find impossible to talk about until they are really sure of you.

3. Why questions are important

Asking the right questions at the right time can be a very powerful intervention. Used well, questions can enable people to:

- Look at current experiences, behaviours and feelings more closely.
- Examine something they had previously overlooked or ignored.
- Clarify attitudes and opinions.
- Become more aware of areas where they need more information.
- Feel valued because they have been asked to contribute.

Helpers may find them useful when they:

- Need some specific information.
- Hope to encourage the service user to participate.
- Want to demonstrate respect for the other person's opinions.
- Need to assess the extent of knowledge.
- Hope to direct attention to a particular behaviour, experience or feeling.
- Need to understand something more clearly.
- Wish to test out the accuracy of their perceptions.

Exercise 20

In groups of three

Take it in turns to play the part of helper, interviewer and observer. Interview each other for approximately 10 minutes. The observer will provide feedback on:

- Use of questions.
- Use of empathy, i.e. responding.
- Listening and attending skills.

Challenging

1. What it is

The helper has two tasks:

1. to understand the world as it appears to another;
2. to facilitate change in line with the other's values and wishes.

Challenging describes a series of verbal techniques used to promote change by the development of learning which in turn will result in new behaviour. Whereas empathy seeks to directly reflect the other person's world, challenges do not. They are arrived at by careful listening and observation on the part of the helper, who then offers a different perspective for the other person's consideration.

The underpinning values of respect and genuineness are very important here because the helper is dealing with material which may as yet be unknown to the listener (e.g. Johari's window). There is usually some good reason why people are unaware; it may be that certain things feel too painful to face or that they may trigger off conflicts which would be extremely threatening.

By challenging, the practitioner is engaging someone directly in a number of ways by:

- Making explicit issues which previously have been implicit and unclear.
- Promoting the ownership of problems, strengths and needs.
- Highlighting the use of evasions and self deceptions.
- Exploring the causes of inertia and inaction.
- Providing feedback on the use being made of the helping relationship.
- Using the relationship with the helper to examine habitual ways of relating which may have a direct bearing on the management of problems.

Absolutely basic to the idea of challenge is that change is a real possibility for everyone. It is a belief which obviates the need for pity and makes the difficult task of working on painful problems hopeful and purposeful.

2. *Different types of challenge*

Challenges include a number of verbal tactics which invite the other person to review, reconsider and, possibly, move from their present position. Just as questions can be seen as an invitation to explore, so a challenge indicates the possibility of change. The following strategies all fall into the category of challenge. They include summary, information giving, self sharing, confrontation, immediacy and what Egan calls 'advanced empathy'.

Summary
Summaries are sometimes seen as half way between empathic reflections and a challenge. This is because although they are firmly based on what has been said, helpers are selective about what is relayed back, using their judgement about what seems to be the central issues. Like other challenges, this more focused picture provides an opportunity for review and development.

To summarise well the helper must have listened not only to the words which were spoken but also to the feeling, tone, perspective, prospect, central identification and theme (Kennedy 1977). Summarising is frequently used in everyday speech. For example, good chairpersons at meetings often summarise and reflect. No doubt this will be a familiar technique to you but it is one which requires skill. In work within a helping relationship summarising can be particularly useful:

- At the beginning of a session, to review the progress to date and maybe to raise what was of major concern last week, e.g. 'Last week you were feeling very concerned because you were without any help in the house and you had real problems just coping with basic necessities like eating, getting to bed and dressing.'
- At the end of the session to review the content of that session.
- When a particular session seems to be rambling and unclear.
- When people are needing help in establishing their priorities.
- When a review of the work accomplished so far would be useful.

Exercise 21

In pairs

- Take it in turns to play the role of helper while the other person discusses an issue related to their practice as a community practitioner for between 5 and 10 minutes. The helper should use a mixture of empathy, questions and, when it seems appropriate, summary to highlight the key issues presented.

N.B. It would be useful to tape the session (using either video or audio) so that each partner has the opportunity to identify and evaluate the use of skills.

- The helper should ask their partner whether:

  - their summary included the critical issues;
  - the way in which it was expressed was clear and to the point;
  - any omissions or misconceptions should be noted and the reasons for them carefully discussed.

Advanced empathy

Gerard Egan uses this phrase to describe 'hunches' that the practitioner may develop based upon an exploration of the problem situation and the understanding this affords. In using this skill helpers offer their perceptions to help someone gain a new perspective which may lead to a more successful management of problems. These perceptions are not plucked from the air but are the result of attentive listening.

Despite the label, little known outside counselling circles, it is a skill quite commonly used by helpers. The three examples below illustrate its use.

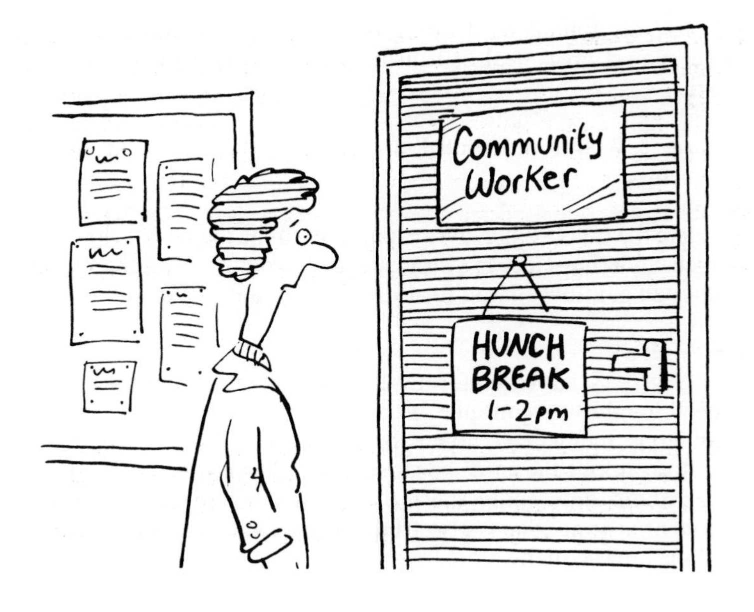

Example 1
Pat, a 40-year-old mother of two, has just returned home following rehabilitation after a road traffic accident.

Pat. Yes, I have done some of the exercises but I'm feeling so tired. I thought when I got home I'd feel better.

Helper. So although you are glad to be home maybe it also puts some extra pressure on you.

Pat. Yes, once you're back you are expected to carry on as usual.

Here the helper has made explicit what were vague half-expressed messages. These difficulties, having been openly acknowledged, can now be addressed.

Example 2
George is 81 and is recovering from a mild stroke. He talks to his community practitioner about his part in the 1939–45 war, his job as an ambulance driver and his care of his wife who died last year.

George. I don't regret anything that I've done, even if it has been hard at times.

Helper. It sounds as if doing things for people has always given you a great deal of satisfaction. You see yourself as a helper.

George. Well I did, but I'm feeling pretty useless at the moment.

Here the practitioner gives expression to the theme of helping which underlies George's stories. This recognition of change, although painful can lead to adjustments to a new reality.

Example 3
Rita, aged 58, has cared for her elderly mother for many years. She is unable to continue because of chronic asthma. Her mother is living in a home for elderly people and Rita is unhappy about the care she is receiving. At various times she talks about how guilty she feels and wears herself out with frequent visiting. She is also frightened because her attacks of asthma are becoming more frequent.

Helper. I wonder whether your poor health isn't connected with all the upset you've experienced since you've been unable to care for your mother. You have been so worried about her and given yourself such a tough schedule of visiting that your body must be feeling the effects.

Here the practitioner helps Rita make connections between various aspects of her life. Bringing all these issues together helps Rita see that she needs to take action because of the damage she is inflicting on herself and possibly her mother as well.

Exercise 22

In pairs

Take it in turns to be the helper. Each take about 10–15 minutes to discuss ways in which you would like to be able to communicate more effectively with those with whom you work. Identify those areas where you find it difficult to be open; such as sex, money, religion or race. See if you can trace the origins of this reticence. The helper should facilitate this process by using sensitive listening, empathy, questions, summary and advanced empathy.

The work should be reviewed in terms of:

- How the helper facilitated this review.
- What feelings such a review evoked in the interviewee.
- Did you discern any fresh insight that might help you improve your communication.

This last exercise was a demanding one, but very important. We cannot effectively challenge other people unless we accept that personal development and change is both necessary and desirable for helpers as well as for those who receive our services.

Information giving

Information giving may not immediately be perceived as a challenging skill; it sounds fairly neutral, but it is concerned with promoting change.

Example
Janice, 21, has recently suffered a bereavement. Her boy friend, Peter was killed in a motorbike accident 4 months ago.

Janice. I think I'm going mad. . . . I keep hearing Pete's bike pulling up outside our house at night.

Helper. You sound really frightened by that. I wonder if you know that this does sometimes happen to people who have lost someone important to them.

Janice. Oh, perhaps I'm not going mad, then, but . . .

Other examples could include practical information about organisations, benefits or other resources. Information giving differs from advice giving because it does not seek to influence the hearer but offers a better basis from which decisions can be made.

Exercise 23

Individually or in pairs

Think about the way either possession of appropriate information or a lack of it has affected some area of your life. This may be personal or professional.

In groups

Review the areas in which you are commonly responsible for offering information to others. Look at the various ways this information is offered:

- Is it sufficiently clear?, i.e. stated in terms that are meaningful to the recipient.
- Are there possibilities for the recipient to review this information?, e.g. straight repetition, audio/video tapes, diagrams.
- Is it given in reasonable dosages? In other words, is there enough to stimulate but not too much so that it overwhelms?
- How adequately is the impact of the information explored and the possibilities for change elaborated?

The helper is acting as a teacher and basic teaching precepts are important.

- Start where the other person is, i.e. establish the baseline of existing knowledge.
- Express the information in a way which is easy to assimilate.
- Check that this information is seen as relevant to their problem.
- Offer adequate opportunities for review.

Self sharing

The helping relationship is one where one person makes themselves available to another in order to work with them to achieve positive change. It requires an openness on the part of the helper and a willingness to involve themselves in a real way. At times this may require them to disclose aspects of themselves, their lives or feelings, which seem to be relevant to the task in hand.

There are questions we have to ask as helpers before talking about ourselves:

In relation to feelings. Will this provide a useful model?, i.e. will it signal permission to the other person to be more intimate? In some circumstances it could be experienced as the helper demanding attention for their own concerns.

In relation to experiences and behaviours. Is my understanding of a particular common experience sufficiently well advanced that I can offer it to someone without adding to their own burden? It is important that any information offered is for the service of the other person not to relieve the helper.

In relation to beliefs and ideas. Is my desire to open up ideas and offer new perspectives, in order to broaden the options available for action? Am I free from any desire to control or dominate them?

In relation to the working alliance. Is this self disclosure likely to control or increase or diminish our ability to work together?

All these decisions can be difficult and there is no easy rule of thumb for every occasion. When it seems right for the helper to use it, it is important to:

- keep it brief and well focused;
- show its relevance to your work together.

Exercise 24

Individually

Review your current practice. Which are the areas where you have direct personal, as well as professional, experience? In what circumstances would you feel it appropariate to share this with the people with whom you work?

Write a brief example of how you might phrase this self sharing.

Example

You may have had a personal experience of sudden bereavement. The father of David, a 19-year-old, has died suddenly.

David. A little while ago everything seemed as if it would go on forever. Now everything has turned upside down. It's all so black! I don't feel life will ever be the same again.

Helper. No, you're right; it can't be. When something similar happened to me, I found things gradually got better. Although it wasn't the same as before, life did go on; but perhaps you aren't ready to think ahead at present.

Here the helper does not deny the feelings expressed or try to rush ahead to a resolution but, from experience, it does indicate survival is possible.

In pairs

Taking it in turns to be in the helping role, share your experience of completing the previous exercise. Give each other feedback on the way self sharing has been used.

In groups

As an intervention, what are its dangers and advantages? What guidelines would you offer an inexperienced practitioner about the use of self sharing?

Confrontation

In everyday speech this has overtones of aggression and in fact this is a particularly direct form of challenge. It is used when the helper feels that progress is being limited or sabotaged in some way. It requires that the practitioner is able to:

- time the intervention sensitively and appropriately;
- word it in a way which does not sound judgemental or aggressive;
- offer a clear explanation of the evidence on which the confrontation is made.

There are a number of reasons why it may be necessary to confront. They include:

- *Denying the existence of the problem.* Some people resist change on the grounds that everything is all right as it is.

- *Refusing to own the problem.* All the time this is attributed to others it is beyond the control of the person experiencing it, e.g. my wife/husband/father/mother does not understand/love/respect/help me scenario.

- *Perceiving the problem in self-defeating ways.* That is, if people perceive themselves as being victims of their past, incapable of action, trapped by fate, exceptionally fragile or always needing to be in control. (Ellis', 1962, work on irrational beliefs is useful in this context.)

  There are certainly some things which cannot be changed in any situation but it is possible to manage them in a more or less constructive way. Death, disability, desertion, loneliness and poverty are all very real but they can be faced and worked on despite the pain and unfairness they often entail.

- *Relating in ways which compound the problem.* Some people have developed ploys and devices which pattern their dealing with others in a way which offers predictability if not satisfaction. (See Eric Berne's *Games People Play* (1964) and *Sex in Human Loving* (1973).) These often threaten to disable the helping relationship as well as harming other potential sources of support.

Confrontation is necessary when someone is primarily deceiving themselves rather than because they wish to deceive the helper. This has been done as a protection from a reality which cannot be faced. It is only, then, in the context of a supportive relationship that confrontation can be used, otherwise all the old defensiveness will come into play. Sometimes helpers bemoan the fact that despite making very true and helpful observations they are ignored and discarded. This has probably more to do with the appropriateness of the challenge than the accuracy of their observations.

As well as being appropriate, confrontations depend for their helpfulness on the practitioner having faithfully observed the situation and having acquired a perception which, when shared, will offer a new dimension on the problem. This in turn will open up the possibility of change.

Because challenges are concerned with areas of conflict it is important they are based on available strengths rather than weakness. We are much more likely to respond to a recognition of our strengths as a springboard for action than a description of our failings.

Helpers must also be aware that, in the end, a challenge is our perception of a situation influenced by our understandings and values. They may well, from time to time, be mistaken and, even if true, may not have meaning to the person being challenged. All challenges must be made bearing these points in mind. This should prevent us from laying down the law and provide us with a suitable degree of tentativeness in making a challenge.

Exercise 25

Individually

Identify an occasion when you have been confronted:

- How was this done?
- How did you react?
- Were you able to make use of the confrontation?
- Are there any issues around the experience that are still unresolved?
- What can you learn from this which will influence your practice?

In pairs

In turns, discuss the problems you experienced in receiving feedback from others. As helper challenge any observed strength which your partner may be discounting in the management of these situations.

Immediacy

Immediacy is a challenging skill which directly focuses on the relationship or the process which exists between the helper and the other person. It is a powerful intervention because it deals with behaviours, experiences or feelings which are not reported but have been mutually experienced. It therefore has a directness and an authenticity which other challenges may lack.

Example

Jane, 43, suffers from multiple sclerosis. She welcomes the chance to discuss the problems she is experiencing in daily living. If discussion moves to how the situation might be managed more effectively she becomes defensive and accuses the practitioner of 'not understanding'.

Helper. Although you seem to want to tell me about the very real difficulties you have, you seem to resent any discussion of how these might be managed. I just wonder whether you feel that if things were a bit easier I might feel you were OK and stop coming.

Because it is concerned with the interaction it has the effect of both valuing and strengthening the relationship, by acknowledging the importance it has in the eyes of the helper. For many people it is a new experience to be taken seriously let alone being exposed to a discussion of what is going on in the relationship. It therefore has to be used with sensitivity but it can also be a valuable source of learning. The helping relationship is not a conventional, social one and this is nowhere more evident than in the use of immediacy. In everyday life we do not, generally, go around giving people feedback on the quality of our relationships or the nature of our transactions. These two activities are exactly those with which immediacy is concerned and emphasises the a-social nature of the helping relationship.

To use this type of challenge effectively, the practitioner needs to:

- Be sufficiently in touch with their own feelings, as well as those of others, so they can identify what is taking place between them.
- Be able to express this in a way which has meaning for the recipient.
- Be assertive, having sufficient confidence in their ability to use the situation constructively.
- Be open; in other words, having a genuine desire to explore the relationship and receive feedback as well as give it.

Exercise 26

Individually

Think of a situation where you have been aware that something in your relationship with a colleague has been getting in the way of your cooperating fully.

- Identify what it is.
- Write down how this might be expressed to your colleague.

In pairs

Role play the situations which you have worked on in the individual exercise, briefing your partner beforehand about the situation. After each role play is completed ask your partner for feedback on:

- How well you expressed your own feelings about the relationship.
- The delivery of your challenge to the other person about their part in it.
- The feelings they experienced, in role, on receiving it.

Discuss what can be learnt from this exercise about the use of immediacy.

3. How to use challenge

Throughout many of the preceding exercises you have been asked to consider how you would use the various types of challenge. Again it must be emphasised that just as they can be effective in helping the client find new ways of framing their problem, leading to more positive management, so if badly used they can undermine or even terminate useful work.

To conclude, the following points are crucial:

- Always offer challenge as a possibility rather than as an established fact. Helpers have their blind spots; they are not all knowing and they may be wrong.
- Bear in mind people are defensive for a reason and head-on attacks strengthen resistance. Extreme sensitivity and care are needed in making challenges. Challenge strength rather than weakness.
- Challenges are not always necessary, often a combination of empathy and questions will lead to self challenge. This can be an empowering experience and therefore one to be preferred.

- If the practitioner finds they are frequently using challenge and obtaining compliance rather than cooperation, something is wrong. The practitioner needs to examine his or her motivation.
- Practitioners are only entitled to challenge if they, too, are willing to both challenge themselves and to be challenged by others.

Conclusion

The introduction suggested that these skills would not be new to most community practitioners. What this review hopes to provide is a sharper recognition of each skill, leading to a more conscious and effective use of them in community practice.

There are no firm rules about when and where each skill is most useful, but Egan (1990) does suggest that the skills of empathy and questioning are essential at the beginning of a relationship to enable the people to tell their story. The skills of challenge Egan places next in the process, at the point at which the person is developing new ways of viewing their problems as a preparation for embarking upon problem-management activities. Certainly the skills of challenge will only be effective in a relationship where the person receiving help feels heard, valued and accepted. This will usually be built upon careful attending and listening, empathy and a sensitive use of questioning.

For most community practitioners these skills will form a part of their professional repertoire. They are not primarily counsellors, but their work can be greatly enhanced by the development of counselling skills. Far from distracting from the main focus of their work it enables them to define difficulties more clearly, understand the problem as it is experienced by those concerned and develop treatment plans which work because they are rooted in the service user's reality.

References

Berne, E. (1964) *Games People Play – the Psychology of Human Relationships*. Harmondsworth: Penguin.

Berne, E. (1973) *Sex in Human Loving*. Harmondsworth: Penguin.

Egan, G. (1990) *The Skilled Helper: a Systematic Approach to Effective Helping* (4th edn). California: Brooks/Cole.

Ellis, A. (1962) *Reason and Emotion in Psychotherapy*. New Jersey: Lyle Stuart.

Fong, M. and Cox, B. G. (1983) Trust as an underlying dynamic in the counselling process: how clients test trust. In Dryden, W. (ed.) (1989) *Key Issues for Counselling in Action*. London: Sage.

Kennedy, E. (1977) *On Becoming a Counsellor – a Basic Guide for Non-professional Counsellors*. Dublin: Gill and Macmillan.

Luft, J. and Ingham, H. (1979) In Wayne P. R. *et al. Techniques for Effective Communication*. New York: Addison Wesley.
Rogers, C. R. (1961) *On Becoming a Person*. Boston: Houghton Miffin.

Chapter 7

The helping process

Mary Ashwin

Assessment and programme planning in the community

We have reviewed something of the very complex nature of the helping relationship and the different ways, both verbal and non-verbal, in which helpers may work within it. This section looks at the helping activity as a whole, set in an organisation framework, with clear limitations of both time and resources.

The community practitioner may come from a number of professional backgrounds, each with some specific type of intervention aimed at problem management. The specific therapeutic input will, therefore, vary but this section will look at a range of techniques which are basic to every helping relationship.

Each contact, whatever the duration, can be seen as being made up of three phases, all with specific tasks. These will be looked at in turn. They consist of:

1. The beginning, negotiating phase

This section will consider the early stage of the relationship from referral, through the initial contact and assessment to the reaching of a working agreement. This will be preceded by a brief consideration of the ethical issues which are common to all helpers.

2. The middle, working phase

This section looks at the ways of making all inputs as productive as possible. It includes the setting of objectives, implementing action plans and programme monitoring.

3. The terminal, withdrawing phase

This will examine the meaning of endings, the process of evaluation and a consideration of where learning should have occurred.

The beginning, negotiating phase

Ethics in the helping process

The readers of this book are, no doubt, very conscious that as professional helpers we each have professional codes of conduct to which we adhere. Any infringement of this will, rightly, be subject to professional and legal sanctions. We will, therefore, only look at the aspect which applies in the broadest sense across professional boundaries, that of offering ourselves, in the role of helper, to another person who requires our services.

The reason for any helping relationship becoming a matter for ethical concern is because of the structural inequality which exists in it. The helper is in a position of power and those who are helped in a position of relative vulnerability. In extreme cases the feeling of potency this may give the helper and the masochistic pleasure of submission and dependence this may offer the recipient provide the emotional backcloth to many newspaper scandals.

Most professional people avoid open violation of their codes of practice. When they do occur the most common infringements consist of exploitation and breaches of confidentiality (in itself a form of exploitation). The exploitation may entail of extracting unfair financial advantage, sexual misconduct or emotional abuse. The last is often difficult to prove and is, perhaps, the most common. It can even occur without any evil intention on the part of the helper. For this reason we shall consider the nature of the inequality which exists and the implications this has for practice. It prevails, very obviously, in four main areas; that of knowledge, information, expertise and command of resources.

The imbalance of knowledge

Professionals are usually operating in a familiar situation for which they have had specific training and about which they have a good deal of specialised knowledge. In contrast, the recipients of help are suddenly plunged into a new and frightening world where many familiar day-to-day activities have been disrupted or, possibly, lost. This disparity, although obvious, can be overlooked as inevitably we become desensitised by the familiarity of our work.

Imbalance of information

Referral procedures vary but inevitably the community practitioner has some information about the newly referred person while the referred person usually has very little about the helper. This all adds to the feeling of being known about while being relatively unknowing. This again is guaranteed to emphasise the power differential between the two.

Imbalance of expertise

Because of the nature of the situation the practitioner is, usually, equipped with special skills which have value in the problem situation in which the person is involved. Many of the skills which recipients may have spent their lives perfecting will, in these new situations, be irrelevant. While needing and often gratefully accepting the skills of the helper, the recipient is often placed in a dependent position.

Command of resources

The final cornerstone of the practitioner's power is based upon his or her ability to generate and recruit resources. Helpers may also block access to resources as they consider appropriate. Professional integrity in such a situation is clearly of vital importance.

There are certain practices which can ensure that the person being helped is not subject to any abuse as a result of this imbalance of power, which, although inevitable, may be used positively or negatively. These practices include:

- Ensuring that service users are aware of why help is being offered and what the nature of that help will be.
- Making the limits of confidentiality clear.
- Offering help in a way which respects the rights of the individual to cooperate or not.
- Providing help which is in accord with the value system of the recipient.
- Minimising gaps in knowledge, information, expertise and command of resources by the use of collaborative, consultative and cooperative approaches which offer a valued and positive role to the recipient of help.

The referral

The people with whom we work do not appear by magic; they are either referred by some person or agency or they refer themselves. It is easy to overlook this stage of the helping process, as if it is not really part of it at all but merely a trigger which precipitates it. In fact the referral is a matter of importance to both the practitioner and the person referred. Both will be powerfully influenced by the source and the nature of the referral.

For the person referred

Influential factors at this stage will include:

- *The knowledge they have of the referral and the reasons given for it having been made.*

It may be assumed that correct information has been given to the referee and that it has been given in a way which is readily absorbed. This is often not the case. When people are experiencing high anxiety their ability to register and process information is impaired and communications are often influenced by the impact of this anxiety.

- *The way in which the referral has been experienced.*

This can be positive, providing access to appropriate and desirable expertise and resources. Sometimes it may be seen as a fobbing-off process, an indirect form of rejection by the person making the referral. Another negative reaction might be that it involves yet more unwelcome and potentially damaging interference into a problem that is already hard enough to bear.

For the helper

Other factors may be at work which are equally influential. Referrals are not all received neutrally and are often awarded high or low priority or greeted with greater or lesser enthusiasm. The factors influencing the practitioner will be:

The emotional impact of the referral
This will be the result of data such as the age, sex and social grouping of the person referred, as well as the obvious influence of the nature of the problem for which they have been referred.

The anticipated usefulness of the helper's intervention
Past experience powerfully affects present responses and this is true of the helping process. It allows experienced workers to make judgements more confidently and assess priorities more expertly. It can also lead to mistakes based on inaccurate or incomplete data. Generally, however, if the helper sees that the referral offers an

opportunity for the appropriate use of their particular form of expertise, they are more likely to respond positively.

The source of the referral

At the referral stage, practitioners are aware of themselves as a part of a therapeutic network, which may sometimes be faulty or incomplete, sometimes adequate and well resourced. Their feelings towards other members of this network will affect the way in which they receive the referral. All colleagues are not accepted equally and our opinion of their professionalism and the quality of their judgements are varied, as are our perceptions of their motivation to refer. A referral from one colleague may appear like a vote of confidence in your expertise and a reinforcement of your professionalism; from another it may be experienced as emotional and professional dumping, causing resentment and a sense of exploitation with a heightened sense of fatigue.

The referral phase, then, is one which greatly influences both the referred and the helper as they embark together on a shared enterprise. This has been explored at some length precisely because many attempts to understand difficulties encountered in a relationship often do not reach back far enough in seeking their source.

Exercise 1

Individually, in pairs or in groups

Review:

- The way in which you receive referrals.
- The way in which you prioritise them.
- The support you receive in processing them.

How do these processes affect your practice?
Are there any changes that you would like to make?

Establishing a working relationship

The method of contact, the preparation of the recipient and the amount of time available for a particular contact are often outside the control of the practitioner. The helper's first opportunity to influence the future outcome will often be on their initial visit. The practitioner's task of assessment is often emphasised at this point but the process is mutual. Everyone concerned in the first meeting will be involved in appraisal. Everything the helper does will be noted and interpreted; both verbal and non-verbal behaviour, e.g. if, where and when you sit down, whether or not you accept an offered drink, what you are wearing, how much, if anything, you write down etc.

The helper's tasks in this situation are to:

- Present themselves as competent, purposeful professionals with specific areas of expertise.
- Explain the purpose of the contact.
- Demonstrate their willingness to listen.
- Convey reasonable warmth.
- Establish the extent and limitations of confidentiality where this is an issue.

Identifying the problem

Referrals will vary in the degree of explicit problem definition they include. The helper's task is to move beyond the initial diagnosis of medical or social pathology towards an understanding of the effect that the diagnosis has on the lives of those on whom it impinges.

The helper's task is to collect the relevant data which will give them a clear understanding of the meaning of the problem. There will be five main sources of information:

- The person seen as needing help.
- Others closely involved.
- The practitioner's observations.
- Other professionals.
- Available data.

The person who has been referred

In many circumstances the person's view of the situation may be close to that of the referee. This is by no means a universal experience, however. Service users may disagree with the way in which the problem has been perceived in terms of:

Ownership
They may see the difficulty as belonging elsewhere, e.g. as a failure of service provision or family cooperation.

Intensity
Although there may be a willingness to admit the problem, they may feel that the degree of difficulty associated with it has been either under or over stated.

Centrality
A problem may be recognised as real but still be seen as having only marginal importance and its solution or management therefore be of very low priority.

In all three cases the helper has either to withdraw or redefine the problem in a way which is meaningful. If this can be done its resolution will be seen as having value and work towards that end worthwhile.

Another problem commonly encountered at this stage may be gaining contact with the person who has been referred. Once through the door other barriers may be encountered. These may be communication barriers, resulting from physical or mental disability, or they may be social barriers erected by others on grounds of age, either youth or senescence or because of their position within the family or social group. The chief concern for the practitioner must be: establishing whether the referral was appropriate or not, and, if appropriate, ensuring the possibility of future contact. (It is important to find out how power is allocated within the family or social group and work with this in mind.)

Others closely involved

Sometimes the helper is told more than one story on the first visit. Each takes place in the same background and the people have common names but there any similarity ends. These differing perceptions are not unusual but they can perplex practitioners as they try to arrive at a clearer identification of the problem.

One way of dealing with this is to see both stories as essentially 'true', e.g. the truth according to Mrs Brown may be 'I really need very little help, we manage very well, I don't think there is really any need for you to see me.' The truth according to Mr Brown may be 'I'm getting worn out, I have to do everything now and I'm not well myself. . . .' They may both be true because, within the context of their particular relationship, the level of dependency may be quite acceptable to Mrs Brown while her husband is feeling overwhelmed by it. So while, perhaps, initially confusing, these different stories tell the practitioner a great deal about the nature of their relationship and the quality of communication within it.

Many of the divergencies between stories centre around behaviour, particularly behavioural difficulties like 'He can't get dressed on his own'. Two common sources of inaccuracy are:

Familiarity
When people know each other well they may be unreliable because they perceive only expected behaviour.

Custom
People fall into routines and assume that the behaviour involved in that routine indicates the full range of behaviour of which the other person is capable.

When meeting other people, then, the helper is:

- Listening to their account of the problem.
- Assessing what is their part in the problem situation.
- Assessing what their contribution will be to the problem management
  - The acceptability of that support to the other person.
  - The reliability of their support if offered.
  - The degree of support available, i.e. in terms of time/effort/frequency.
  - The nature of support they would offer, especially whether this would be of an enabling or controlling kind.

The practitioner's observations

These begin as you drive or walk to a particular street; already the location will have alerted you to the possible social grouping of the person you are visiting. The initial meeting at the door, the quality of welcome and the extent to which you are allowed to penetrate into the house (i.e. sitting room, kitchen or bedroom etc.) will all provide you with an even richer fund of information about the problem's social context. You will have made guesses about the degree of affluence, probable life-style, and started to calculate whether the environment will exacerbate or minimise the problem outlined in the referral.

Exercise 2

Individually or in groups

- Make a checklist of the significant factors you would hope to observe when you are visiting someone for the first time.
- Think about how you would interpret this information, e.g. how would you interpret such data as a broken window?
- How would this influence your approach to the problem situation?

If in a group

- Compare the way in which you have interpreted various observations:

- Are there areas of disagreement?
- Can you think of exceptions?

No doubt you will have generated quite a list of significant factors. Because of the very richness of the situation the observer may suffer from a number of disadvantages which will impair the accuracy of their impressions.

Prior information
Referrals may influence the focus of the observations made. These very real difficulties should lead us to be suitably *tentative* in our interpretation of observations made in first encounters. Where possible it is useful to check out both our observations and interpretations with another community practitioner. Another safeguard is to discuss the situation with a practitioner who is able to challenge our assumptions.

Overload
There may be just too much to take in all at once.

Personal bias
Observers tend to see what they expect to see (e.g. liking often produces a 'halo' effect).

Atypical behaviour
People's behaviour may change considerably in the presence of an unknown professional.

The actions of helpers
Their normal professional activities may interfere with, and alter, characteristic behaviour.

Pressure
The need to keep a schedule may result in the helper ignoring significant events.

Other professionals

Multi-disciplinary teams offer a broad range of ideas and expertise. The helper may well be able to draw on considerable data which has already been assembled by others, to help in a more efficient identification of the problem. Sometimes, however, the very strength of the community team can produce the negative effect of outnumbering and intimidating an individual or their family.

It is important that at this early stage of the relationship a two-way flow of information is established so that, as the practitioner gathers information of someone's world, so they gain information about the helping services. It is particularly important that they know basic information about who is involved, what are their special contributions to the problem-management activities and how they relate to each other and the service user.

Available data

Community practitioners are usually more privileged than the people with whom they work, in that they have ready access to a fund of information. They will include:

Library services
These are offered by social services departments, hospitals, universities, polytechnics and colleges. Local authority libraries also offer valuable services.

Specialist library information services
These include such libraries as the Kings Fund Library offering information on health care issues or The National Children's Bureau Library on the wide field of child care.

General information services
National agencies like the Citizen's Advice Bureau have well developed information systems which are available to both helpers and service users.

Organisations dealing with special categories of need
A useful handbook in this connection is the Charities Handbook which is published annually and is available in the reference section of most libraries. Many of these societies offer very valuable information, advice and in some cases a national or regional network of support groups.

The helper has a responsibility to know as much as possible about a problem situation. Research findings have in general been under utilised by helpers. In the section on 'talking to people' the skill of information giving was discussed; it presupposes that the helper will have done the necessary homework.

After all these sources of information have been explored the practitioner may well find that the problem has been identified very differently by different people or groups. The helper's task will be to make these differences explicit and, where possible, reconcile the differing perspectives.

Collecting information

Having identified the problem area, the practitioner then has to assemble, with everyone else concerned, much more precise data about the problem situation on which to base any action plans. The large amount of information gathered in the initial contact is not discarded but it is subjected to close scrutiny in case unwarranted assumptions have been made.

This stage of the helping process is often described as 'assessment'. This is somewhat confusing, since, as we have seen, assessment begins as soon as the practitioner and the service user meet and it is mutual. It also continues throughout the whole period of contact – called variously assessment, monitoring or evaluation depending on the part of the process in which they are engaged. To avoid this confusion, Brechin and Liddiard (1981) preferred to call it evaluation throughout. The traditional terminology will be used here, but basic skills required for each of the three phases are identical. The two basic skills involved are those of observation and various types of questioning.

Before looking at these in more detail there are two aspects of any assessment that cannot be ignored, these are *reliability* and *validity*.

Reliability
This refers to the stability of results which can be obtained from any particular measurement. For instance, will the results of any measurement vary widely depending on the time or place in which they were taken? Some measurements are easier to arrive at than others, leaving less room for individual variations, e.g. it is easier to measure mobility than life satisfaction. Reliability can be improved by training assessors so that methods of testing and interpreting are standardised.

Validity
This refers to the extent to which a test measures what it is supposed to measure. Many people find exams very disabling and would claim that it is not their knowledge being tested but their exam technique (or lack of it!). Sometimes practitioners' results reflect more about the degree of cooperation, concentration or the person's desire to please than a precise measurement of a particular skill.

Both these aspects have to be taken into account when analysing the results of any data collection. The skills of assessment will now be examined.

Observation

Some of the limitations of the practitioner as an observer have already been suggested and the important distinction made between observation and interpretation, i.e. the difference between what you actually see and what you make of this observation.

There are two main types of observation, and many community practitioners are involved in both. They are:

- Structured observation, in which the practitioner has already selected the items which are to be observed. They are often used in clinical situations where precise information over a prescribed field is required.
- Unstructured observation. Here the observer sets out to discover as much as possible about a situation in order to understand it.

Structured observations are useful when comparisons are required, e.g. Mrs Brown walked along a passage unaided yesterday; can she do the same today? They are not only helpful in keeping a record of performances but also in making comparisons between performances in difficult environments. How does Mrs Brown's performance at the day centre compare with her performance at home? Because they follow the same format each time they are easy to analyse, although, of course, their value will depend upon the items included in the observation checklist.

Unstructured observations were discussed earlier; their main strength lies in their ability to cover a wide range of experience. For this reason they are very subjective since the observer will be forced to be selective because of the sheer quantity of detail. Many community practitioners find it helpful to adopt a semi-structured approach in which they keep in mind a pre-specified checklist of items which are seen as important. If you completed the exercise earlier you will have already written an observational checklist.

All observations are valuable because they are first-hand experiences which are not subject to the bias of any received anecdotes. In the problem-management situation they have a key place in identifying the strengths in the people with whom you will work and the environment in which it will take place.

Exercise 3

Individually or in groups

In your current practice review how your structured and unstructured observations are recorded.

- *In structured observations.* Do the observational criteria cover the areas which you think are crucial? What changes would you like to make, if any?
- *In unstructured observation.* Is the space offered for unstructured observation adequate? What opportunities are there for charting changes and making comparisons?

Various types of questioning

Apart from what we see for ourselves we are dependent upon the reports of others for information. This includes both written and spoken information. There has already been some discussion of the best way to frame questions and clearly this is relevant whether they are spoken or written. Because interviewing is more commonly used than written questionnaires, this section will briefly review the different types of interview and their advantages and drawbacks.

Structured interview

This is rarely used in community practice unless the practitioner is engaged in some special study. It consits of a set of standardised questions, which are always offered asked in the same order. They are a useful vehicle:

- when information about facts rather than feelings is required;
- when comparisons are needed between different respondents;
- if properly used are less suspect to interviewer bias;
- simpler to record.

Their disadvantages are:

- questions may be interpreted in various ways making comparisons rather involved;
- no room is allowed for development or exploration as answers are sometimes incomplete and therefore misleading;
- some questions may have no relevance to the interviewee so that answers are meaningless.

Semi-structured interview

This is generally more widely used. In this type of interview the same core questions are always asked, but they may be reworded if something is not clear. It is also possible in this looser interview to add other questions which arise out of the interviewee's responses.

They have the advantages of a structured interview that answers to core questions can be compared, but because of the greater flexibility are more open to interviewer bias, both in the interaction itself and in its recording.

Focused interviews

The interviewer begins a focused interview having identified a list of issues that should be covered, but the way in which they are covered is not specified. Because they are more conversational in tone they encourage respondent participation. They are useful because:

- they allow a much deeper consideration of topics;
- they allow the interviewee to raise issues which may have been overlooked;
- they allow exploration of beliefs and attitudes.

The drawbacks are:

- bias is more likely because of the flexibility afforded to both interviewer and respondent;
- interview control may be more testing for the interviewer;
- successful interviews will be those where rapport has been established, therefore perceived differences may cause less favourable responses;
- time consumption is high, both for the interview itself and the subsequent recording of the information gained from it.

Open-ended interviews

In this type of interview the interviewer raises the topic to be discussed and allows the interviewee to develop it in their own way. The advantages of this approach are:

- the interviewer does not contaminate the interviewee with his/her own thinking;
- the interviewee has space to develop the topic in a way which has personal meaning;
- the material will be much 'richer' and may address very personal and sensitive issues.

The drawbacks are:

- the interviewer needs considerable skill, in both obtaining the information and interpreting it;
- it will be difficult to analyse (see above);
- if comparisons with other interviewees are needed these will be hard to make.

Very often in community practice the use of very formal interviewing techniques is limited. However, an understanding of the effects of pre-planning and structure is important. When time is such a precious commodity the most efficient ways of obtaining vital information has to be a matter of importance.

Exercise 4

Individually. For consideration

Is there any way in which you could improve the structure of your interviews without damaging the rapport between yourself and the service user?

Analysing data to plan for change

The scope and detail of any information-gathering exercise will depend upon the use for which it is intended. For example, if it is used simply to determine access to a particular resource it will be limited and sharply focused on a number of relevant issues. This section addresses its use as the basis of a problem-management programme. It will include four main ways in which data can be used to generate treatment plans. They are the examination of causes, an appraisal of current functioning, a review of change possibilities and proposals for problem management.

What is causing the problem?

Community practitioners need to define problems creatively if they are to be constructively addressed. If, for instance, one accepts a condition, like blindness, as the 'problem' then very little can be done about it. It is worth, then, making a distinction between situations which can be cured or radically improved and those which have to be accepted as part of that person's reality. Drawing the line between passive acceptance and realistic acceptance is not in itself easy and is something which has to be addressed on an individual basis. On the whole, however, it is better to see what is unchangeable as the reality rather than as the problem.

If we exclude from our consideration problems which are immediately susceptible to direct treatment, there are a number of other factors to be considered which may offer some room for real improvements. They include:

The management of the problem
Although it is not always possible to change the problem situation,

it is often possible to manage it in more constructive ways. For example, incontinence may be irreversible but the way in which it is managed will very much determine its social consequences. Often it will be the social consequences which constitute a very painful aspect of the condition.

The environment

Many problems are exacerbated and, in some instances, caused by the social conditions in which a person may be operating. There is truth in the saying 'There are no disabled people, only disabling environments.' Studies of institutions from the 1960s onward show how vulnerable we all are to environmental pressure. Any attempts to understand the causes of problems must include these factors.

Personal adjustment

As studies of older people show, there is no direct connection between dependency and handicap. So much will depend upon the attitude of the person who is experiencing a difficulty. Seligman's (1975) work on 'learned helplessness' emphasises the damaging and potentially deadly effects of lost hope.

Community helpers will be very conscious that this whole area of personality and relationships may be a source of difficulty. (Hopefully they will be helped by the section on 'talking to people'.) To further complicate matters, the need for readjustment is not necessarily located in the person referred with the 'problem'.

Social support systems

These are again a manifestly crucial area and deficient or malfunctioning support systems quickly breed any number of problems. The section on groups and working with families may offer some ideas of how such causes may be identified and constructively addressed.

What is happening now?

The analysis of the current situation will produce three useful types of information. It will give a clear understanding of the problem, a baseline of current performances and some awareness of the available strengths which can be used in problem management to offset the needs which will also exist.

Understanding the problem

Once the problem situation has been identified necessary data about the problem will include answers to the following:

- Where is the problem located? (i.e. a person, family or group?)
- How frequently does it occur?
- When does it occur? With whom? Where?
- At what time of day? How long does it last?
- How controllable is it?
- What degree of difficulty does it involve?
- What kind of event precipitates it?
- What are the consequences of the problem?
- Who shares in these consequences?

This systematic review of every possibility will ultimately be a great time saver since it is easy to misunderstand the nature of problems; by the time the community practitioner meets them they have developed their own mythology.

A baseline of current performances

Once a situation is experienced as problematic it is important to analyse the different behaviours which exist within it. A useful checklist of questions is:

- What are the current patterns of behaviour?
- Is the problem seen in terms of desirable behaviours which are not occurring or occurring too infrequently?

If so:

Do the individuals have the necessary skills?
Are there any approximations to the desired behaviour?
What seems to be the main difficulties which block the desired performances?

- Is the problem seen in terms of undesirable behaviours which are causing disruption and/or distress?

If so:

What degree of control do individuals have over these behaviours?
What conditions makes this behaviour more likely to occur?
Are there other conditions/behaviours which perpetuate this behaviour?

These questions will be answered using a combination of observation and questioning. Very often helping agencies themselves issue checklists of behaviours which fall into these two categories;

for example, dependency measures for elderly people. However, what is important is to identify together the behaviours which are central to the distress experienced. Completion of a skills checklist will only provide information about functioning, and this will require sensitive interpretation if the central causes of distress are to be identified.

Strengths and needs

Any problem analysis should provide those involved with information about the positive aspects of the situation. This is important since, as we discussed earlier, successful changes are based on strengths. Deficits or needs have to be considered but with a view to their eventual management rather than as a vital component of the programme structure.

The strengths in the situation will be located in the individual, their family or social group, the community, the helper and their organisation.

- *The individual.* This includes all the things that people are able to *do*, as well as those attitudes and beliefs which motivate and maintain them.

- *Family or social group.* This includes any of those people who are in contact with the service users, and who are willing to offer practical and emotional support.

- *Community.* The strength of the community consists of all the resources which may be used in problem management. These include voluntary and statutory social service agencies and informal neighbourhood networks.

- *The helper.* This consists of all the skills, information and concern which the helper brings to the situation. This in turn will be supported by all the contacts and services which exist within their organisational framework.

The needs in the situation consists of all those aspects which require attention and are often stated in terms of 'problems', although they can be seen, more productively, as constituting targets for change.

Taken together these three types of analysis should provide important clues as to how the problem situations can be managed more effectively.

What is the potential for change?

The potential for change will be largely determined by the following factors:

The commitment of those involved in effecting change
Problems tend to be attended by tiredness and depression and the practitioner often has to act as the primary change agent. Hope and optimism are valuable attributes which the practitioner can bring to the problem situation, offering an experience of problem management and a range of specialist skills. This enthusiasm may well prove contagious even if the initial response is discouraging.

The willingness to take reasonable risks
Another common response to stress is to cling on to what is predictable and known in a threatening situation. One of the practitioner's tasks may be to enable people to abandon fixed patterns of behaviour that lock them into a problem situation.

Creative thinking
A problem with an easy solution is not really a problem at all. Most problem situations are not simple and their management requires creative thinking. Nonconformity, flexibility, curiosity and persistence are all important in finding ways around knotty problems.

No change is achieved without cost and although this is not always openly acknowledged people's behaviour tends to show that they are, at some level, aware of this. Because of the costly nature of change it is important to consider:

- Who are seen as responsible for any proposed changes?
- What is the balance between the change costs and change benefits for all those concerned?
- How much change is required before the situation will be experienced as improving?

A useful exercise can be drawing up a balance sheet with those concerned, listing the costs and benefits of each proposed change.

Where would be a good place to begin?

The outcome of problem analysis should be an indication of what the key issues are which require attention:

- A recognition of the behaviours that are perpetrating the problem situation.

- Some sense of priority in terms of the impact of these issues, e.g. someone who is exhausted by pain, is unlikely to be able to think positively about anything other than its possible relief.
- An appreciation of the strengths which can be utilised in order to support the change process.
- A shared understanding of what would constitute positive change – requiring some vision of possible improvement.

Applied to a particular problem situation, this information should help the practitioner and all those involved agree upon a prime target for change, offering the best rewards for the investment made.

Reaching a working agreement

In an ongoing relationship some form of contract will be established between the practitioner and the individual. Although it always exists, it may be implicit or explicit. Often implicit contracts are made up of role expectations which may be reasonable or unreasonable on both sides. The very lack of openness can make problems around the working agreement more difficult to address.

Where explicit contracts do exist they may be informal, verbal contracts or more formal written contracts. These formal contracts are often incorporated into the administration of the helping relationship, with printed forms where both are required to sign, making a firm commitment to certain actions. There is considerable debate about the ethics of such contracts; it is questioned how freely they can be negotiated when the power base between the individual and helper is so unequal, in terms of both choice and control. This tension is evident in the White Paper on Community Care referred to in 'consumer interests and consumer choice' but saw the local authority as the 'customer/purchaser'.

The advantages of a contract are that it makes expectations explicit, provides a clear plan for action, offers a criterion for determining success or failure. The necessary information which has to be included, if a contract is to perform these useful functions, are:

Who is involved?
In a community-based picture it can become a real issue for practitioners to know how far they can formalise informal and family support without damaging relationships.

Time
This includes discussion about the duration and the frequency of any activities.

What has been established as a target for change? (i.e. the goal)
This in turn will have been based upon some consensus about the nature of the problem.

What is the plan for effecting change? (i.e. the objective)
Each step towards the goal should be spelt out, even if they are later modified. This demonstrates the realistic nature of the plan.

What are the tasks?
The task to be completed should be included in the contract, clearly described, showing how they relate to the agreed goal, as well as who will be responsible, within a specified time frame.

Levels of performance
Although it is hard to specify this too closely, without some attempt to give qualitative as well as quantitative guidelines the contract will have little sense.

What will constitute 'success' or 'failure'?
In other words, some indication of the behaviour which will indicate that the goal has been reached.

What is the status of the contract?
What are the rights of all parties in the event of any failures to keep to the agreement outlined? This includes shared information about review or complaint procedures.

Setting goals and objectives

Goals and objectives have been mentioned as part of the shared understanding that should be present in a working agreement. Mager (1974) has written very clearly on both the nature of goals and the setting of objectives.

Goals

To be clear a goal has to define a performance which can be seen to have been achieved. In other words it is about external reality rather than 'internal' states. Mager used the term 'fuzzy' to describe all the real but hard to classify activities. A goal that incorporates words like appreciate, enjoy, understand, or develop will all be fuzzy because they are all about experience rather than outcomes. Clear goals will include words like identify, construct, define and contrast.

An aid for determining whether or not your goal is clear is used by Westamacott; he calls it the 'Hey Dad' test. If you can not show someone what has been achieved when the goal is reached, it's fuzzy.

Examples

Goal
To appreciate English literature.

Hey Dad Test
'Come and see how I've enjoyed this book.'

This is impossible, therefore the goal was fuzzy.

Goal
To outline the plot of *A Winter's Tale*.

Hey Dad Test
'Read my synopsis of *A Winter's Tale*.

Possible, therefore the goal was clear and non-fuzzy.

Objectives

Objectives describe the steps by which the goal is reached. (Egan, 1990, calls them sub-goals.) To be effective objectives have to possess the following qualities – usefully they can be remembered by the anagram SAVE. They will be:

Specific
Just as goals have to be clearly stated, so too objectives have to describe with real precision what each step will involve. They include such information as:

- The nature of the activity.
- Who will be involved.
- To what standard/level it will take place.
- In what conditions it will occur.

Example

Mrs Brown will walk, using a stick, from bedroom to sitting room twice a day.

- Activity – walking.
- Who – Mrs Brown.

- What standards – from bedroom to sitting room (distance); twice a day (frequency).
- What conditions – using a stick.

Adequate
It is important,

- that the objectives are seen as a useful contribution towards meeting the target by all concerned;
- that they fully use the resources of the user, the carer and the helping agency.

Verifiable
That it is possible to check out whether it has been reached or not (see the Hey Dad Test).

Effective
That the objective, when achieved, will make a significant contribution towards managing the problem situation.

Basically the process of goal and objective setting are the same; they are distinguished by the fact that the goal is a statement of intent and the objectives outline each step towards the goal.

The contract-making process

If all parties are clear about the need, content and purpose of a contract, a number of other issues remain.

(a) Who is the author of the contract; is it written by the practitioner and agreed by the service users? Is it written in language that reflects the world of service provider or the service user?
(b) Arising from (a), comprehension may be an issue. There exists a vast difference in word usage. Vocabulary in medical and social service settings is often specialised and distancing.
(c) It is important to test out whether cooperation is genuine or if some parties to the agreement have merely complied to avoid confrontation.
(d) The nature of any reservations or provisos should be made explicit as should any limitations in participation.

The working agreement, then, is concerned with very central issues like power and choice within the helping relationship.

Exercise 5

Individually

Consider how you arrive at working agreements with service users. What are the advantages and disadvantages of your present method of working?

In groups

Brainstorm both the advantages and disadvantages of a formal written contract.

(a) How accurately are these pro's and con's reflected in your practice?
(b) Are there any changes you would like to make in current procedures?

(a) Critically review them in terms of:

- clarity;
- specificity.

(b) Discuss any ethical issues relating to power and freedom which these contracts may provoke.

The middle working phase

The middle phase is characterised by activity; it is concerned with implementing the care plan, maintaining activity and monitering programmes effectiveness. Each of these will now be examined to determine the nature of worker involvement throughout this stage.

Implementing action/care plans

The action plans should be clearly outlined in the objectives; they will all be very different but they will all take account of the needs of the service users, the measure of environmental support and the resources to which the practitioner has access. At the outset of each programme the community practitioner should check the following:

That the plan reflects the strengths, needs and aspirations of the users and/or carers

Any programme will demand some changes on the part of the service user. James Atherton (1986), discussing learning and change, outlines the 'conversion' model used in secular changes (Figure 7.1).

Atherton represents the regenerative framework as the provision of space in which change can occur. This describes precisely the conditions of a planned intervention. The source of the change may be a crisis, a self-realisation of the need to adjust or the new ability to meet the challenge of change because support is now available. 'Conviction' is a recognition that previous behaviour is unproductive and 'renunciation' that the outcomes of that behaviour are not, ultimately, resulting in need fulfilment. The 'new start' constitutes learning new responses and ways of being, resulting in 'new conduct'.

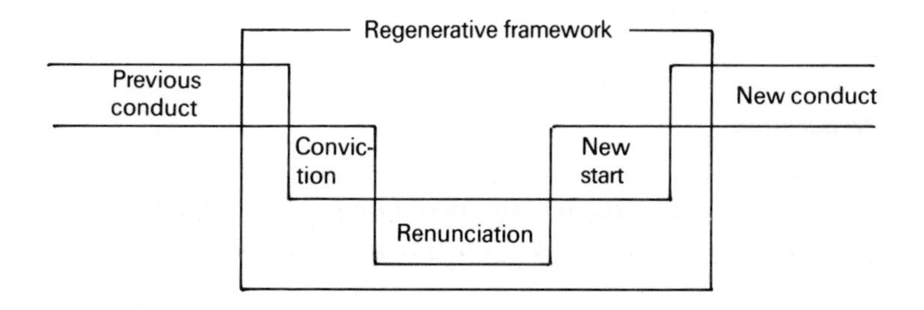

Figure 7.1. Schematic representation of the 'conversion' model of the natural history of threatening learning (Atherton, 1986, p. 157)

The helper in this situation has a number of tasks. They are:

- To alert everyone concerned to the usefulness of the proposed change.
- To clearly state the need which has prompted the action plan.
- To show how the plan will, in theory, manage the problem more effectively.
- To provide a vision of how things will be when the plan is completed.
- To describe the actions which must take place to achieve the desired change.

These actions will be based on a period of shared assessment and will be rooted in shared understandings of both the problem and the actions which will result in positive change.

That the level of support bears direct relationship to the extent of the changes proposed

It is recognised that any learning is accompanied by anxiety. The 'regenerative framework' illustrates some of the demands made on people seriously attempting to learn new behaviours, above and beyond any physical and emotional demands that the programme itself may entail. Familiarity, even if not pleasant, may feel secure.

The helper has three main tasks. They are:

1. Helping the service users/carers prepare for the likely problems which may be encountered during the implementation of the plan.
2. Providing realistic feedback on the actions which form part of the plan.
3. Checking that the necessary resources are in place.

Preparation

Embarking on any new venture involves stress and a degree of risk because it opens up the possibility of failure and that the new state, if achieved, may be worse than the first. For these reasons it is important that the goal is generally recognised as desirable, achievable and capable of making a real contribution towards the management of difficulties.

A useful supportive activity which the community practitioner can initiate is the identification and listing of the forces which will facilitate change and those which will resist it. These lists will be generated, not by the helper but by those who are involved directly in change. They will provide an open and realistic appraisal of the risks and the support for goal attainment. It is a technique known as Force-field Analysis.

Method

- Draw a line upon which you write the goal.
- Above the line write all the forces which are *depressing achievement*. This will include factors inside individuals, their immediate social circle (e.g. family and friends) and their wider environment (e.g. day centre, church, voluntary organisations).
- Below the line, those which are supporting change and helping the person reach their desired performance. Again, include personal, intimate social and wider social, organisational, and cultural factors.

- Having identified both positive and negative factors, score the relative strengths of each of them, e.g. how compulsive is a particular behaviour for the individual. Use a scale of +1 to +3 for positive factors and −1 to −3 for negative factors. Add up estimated +'s and balance against the −'s.
- Devise ways, together, in which the negatives may be weakened and the positives strengthened.
- Review the goal again in the light of this exercise. Even at this late stage it is better to change the goal than expose everyone concerned to a negative learning experience.

Providing feedback

An important aspect of any learning experience is receiving feedback on our performances. Without such feedback, factors that weaken our performances go unnoticed and areas of real strength and expertise are not fully explored. In any helping situation it is important that both users and helpers are able to accept such feedback if plans are to be successful. Useful guidelines for both giving and receiving feedback are:

- Mutual respect and genuineness are essential to avoid negative defensiveness.

In giving feedback:

- Give the feedback as quickly as possible after the behaviour to be discussed.
- Be specific and precise about the behaviour to be addressed.
- Give it in small enough quantities so that the recipient is not overwhelmed.
- Do not say *why* things are wrong but *what* is wrong.
- Choose a time when such feedback is most likely to be heard.
- State clearly how you would like things to be different.

In receiving feedback:

- Accept any comment and check that you have understood before going on to discuss it.
- Acknowledge the other person's right to hold such an opinion.
- Ask for further details if you are still unclear.
- Accept 'facts'.
- Do not accept 'put downs'.

Resource review

At the beginning of any planned work it is important to check that the resources required for the plan to succeed are in place. This will include:

- Checking that services which were already provided are to continue if necessary and that those involved are aware of the action plan.
- Checking that proposed new services are both available and affordable.
- That any gaps in the resources available are recorded and included in the evaluation.
- That practical details such as the timing of provisions the frequency and the quality are known and are acceptable to all concerned.
- That where possible the user has been offered a choice in both the service and its delivery.
- That the full range of both statutory and voluntary services have been used to provide a cost-effective, coordinated and supportive framework for action.

That the administration of the care plan is adequate

The way in which the care plan is administered will vary depending upon the needs of the service user, carers and the local organisation of community care. The assessed needs of the user will determine the complexity of the network. One of the major aims of the NHS and Community Care Act 1990 was to provide a 'seamless service' to its users.

As this vision becomes reality it should result in more clearly defined procedures relating to assessment and care planning and the development of communication systems capable of dealing with the constantly changing information relating to both resources and policies. In turn, these changes should result in the service user experiencing a needs-responsive approach to care planning, a wide choice of services, an increased participation in planning and well publicised mechanisms through which to make representations about both their assessment and the resulting action.

Different agencies will have various systems of care management and at an inter-agency level there will be different patterns of coordination. The community practitioner's responsibility will be:

- To understand the way in which resources are allocated within their agencies (priorities of need and appropriate levels of response).

- To understand the budgetary implications of the care plan (who controls the budget, what are the budget limitations, what constitutes good value for money in terms of problem management and symptom relief).
- To be able to mobilise and coordinate the resources which have been identified in the care plan (this will include a thorough understanding of the agency and inter-agency communications system).
- To manage conflicts that may arise over resource allocations and provision.
- To ensure that service users are aware of their rights and have the necessary information to pursue them.

The position of the community practitioner may not be an easy one in many cases. The last three points indicate areas where there may be disagreements within an agency, between agencies and between users and the agencies providing the services. This will be minimised if a review process is in place and everyone involved is aware of its existence and are kept informed of the dates of the meetings and the extent of their involvement in it. These inter-agency meetings are particularly important in situations where individuals are experiencing severe and challenging difficulties. They are complicated by differences in status, information and input. They benefit from an effective chairperson who is not directly concerned with the service provision and where the users and carers are supported by a community practitioner who has worked with them with some consistency.

Practitioners experiencing situations of conflict need to be clear about the nature of the difficulty:

- Is it a misunderstanding based on faulty communication?
- Is it a genuine conflict, based on a competition for resources or differences in values?
- Is it a personality clash, where people are personally threatened in some way?

If the conflict is based on inadequate communication, the use of attentive listening, empathy and questions to clarify the situation will be effective.

If there is a genuine conflict then it is important to be clear about its exact nature and to not allow it to escalate. Allow a pause if things are becoming overheated and then treat finding a solution as a shared and unifying activity.

If it is a personality clash, try to avoid inflaming it by a lot of talk. If necessary, describe what is going wrong for you and listen to the response. Respect, genuineness and empathy are the best ingredients for overcoming the problem. The unconscious nature of the source of these conflicts make them both hard to control and change. If the conflict seems impossible to solve, it is best to settle for damage limitation by avoiding too much contact and by keeping what contacts there are as well focused and as purposeful as possible.

Summary

By the end of the implementation phase all those participating should be actively involved.

- The action plan should reflect the values and needs of the service user.
- The support system should be adequate to meet the demands of the action plan.
- The roles and tasks of all those participating should be clearly defined.
- The channels of communication should be known and accessible to carers and service users as well as service providers.

Maintaining programmes

Despite careful assessment, care planning and implementation some plans may quickly falter and seem to run out of steam. After the programme has been screened for design defects (this will be dealt with in the following section) the problem may lie in the flagging commitment of users, carers, the helper or other service providers. An understanding of behavioural theory is helpful when motivation seems to be an issue. Behavioural theory rests on the principle that:

- behaviour which is followed by pleasant consequences is likely to be repeated;
- behaviour which is followed by unpleasant consequences will become less frequent.
- behaviour which is no longer reinforced will tend to disappear.

Reinforcement

Rewarding people in behavioural terms is generally associated with activities like praise and attention. Nothing, however, is universally reinforcing so that in the case of a programme faltering it is often worth discussing whether the rewards are sufficient to encourage progress. The goal of the programme may well elicit enthusiasm, but if it is too distant it may not prove a strong enough motivator in the face of fatigue, depression or competing interests. Some goals, although seeming as if they offer positive rewards, may in fact prove negative. One woman, who lived in a residential home for the elderly, found that she lost the close attention of another resident as she became more mobile. Her friend preferred a companion who was dependent and could provide an outlet for her caring needs. What therefore might have been experienced as a pleasurable opening of new possibilities was experienced as a loss of intimacy.

Locating what is reinforcing for a particular person is the real nub of the problem. The sort of questions which might help are:

'What are your main interests or hobbies?'
'What sort of people do you enjoy being with?'
'What makes you happy/relaxed/contented?'
'What would you do if you won the pools?'
'What kinds of things are really important to you?'

Negative reinforcement does not operate in a depriving way, but rather reinforces certain behaviours by linking them to the avoidance of an adverse effect. You are encouraged to buy a railway ticket in order to avoid the disgrace of a criminal record. Helpers often encourage participation in a therapeutic programme by outlining the dangers of inaction.

Punishment

The woman who lost her friend experienced her increased mobility as having been punished; in other words, it resulted in unpleasant consequences and her motivation to persevere with demanding mobilisation routines was, understandably, greatly diminished. This form of punishment was unintentional and could have been avoided if the woman's friend had been helped to see how much more positively she could help by assisting with the therapy.

Most helpers do not like to think that they use punishment to modify behaviour. In practice most of us do, often unconsciously re-enacting our own punishing experiences. The helping relationship, as we discussed earlier, inevitably involves dependence so that the helper's withdrawal of approval, warmth or attention may well be experienced as punishment.

Some limitations of punishment are:

- It does not generate any new learning because it only inhibits a particular behaviour. In contrast, people whose initiative has been rewarded in one area will often go on to develop it in others.

- Because of the unpleasant nature of the experience further learning may be discouraged and potentially useful initiatives dropped.

Extinction

This is the process by which behaviours are often eliminated by lack of either positive or negative reinforcement. Extinction refers to the cessation of both the procedure and the behaviour which decreases and often ceases completely in the face of such withdrawal. In some programmes this can come about unintentionally because the right schedule of reinforcement has not been found.

Forward chaining and backward chaining

Behavioural theory also offers ideas which may be useful if the structuring of the programme is presenting a problem. Chaining and backward chaining involves a detailed task analysis of each step towards a desired goal. The teaching of the target behaviour may begin either from the beginning of a chain of actions (forward chaining) or from the end (backward chaining). In backward chaining the tea may be made, cups put ready and the first step would be pouring out the tea. In forward chaining one might begin by filling the kettle. The choice of these techniques will depend to a large extent on what will prove more reinforcing to the learner.

Patterns of reinforcement

The way in which reinforcement is offered has been exhaustively investigated. Generally reinforcement is most effective if it immediately follows the action. Once established, behaviours are maintained by intermittent reinforcing. An example is the considerable effectiveness of spot-checks as a method of quality control. To be a complete success goal behaviours should be maintained with self-administered, internal reinforcement because they are seen as having real value. This is achieved by fading, the gradual withdrawal of positive reinforcement.

Critical incident analysis

One way of finding out what may be preventing progress proceding successfully is a detailed examination of difficult situations. This involves the description, analysis and role play of difficult incidents in order to prevent recurring patterns of failure by providing new ways of behaving in the problem situation. Priestly *et al.* (1978) support the action replay approach in which people are asked to imagine they are making a film of their own critical incidents. They used an extended version of the 5W–H exercise to elaborate and analyse the incident. *W*ho is involved– *W*hen *W*here *W*hat happened are used in role play preparation and *W*hy and *How* used to analyse the role play.

Two ABC analyses

The skill in all the behavioural techniques is in determining what it is in any planned activity that is experienced as rewarding. There are two methods of analysing behaviour that offer help with this problem, both called ABC.

The first ABC of behavioural work is discussed by Herbert (1985). In this method ABC stands for Antecedents, Behaviours and Consequences.

Example

Antecedent. Mr S. is asked to complete an exercise.

Behaviour. Mr S. says he is too tired.

Consequences. The practitioner spends some time explaining its importance and the possible results of such behaviour.

Such analysis, over time, might lead one to conclude that Mr S. actually received more attention by not involving in the treatment than by exercising. This would offer important clues as to what he experienced as reinforcing and how the practitioner might address the problem more effectively.

The second ABC model is outlined by Tschudi (1977). In this model:

A is the problem
a(1) – the actual state.
a(2) – the desired state.

B is the desirability of the solution
b(1) – the disadvantages of a(1).
b(2) – the advantages of a(2).

C is what prevents movement
c(1) – the advantages of a(1).
c(2) – the disadvantages of a(2).

Example

This could be applied to the woman who lost her friend. The exercise may have gone as follows:

A: the problem	a(1) – can't get out of wheelchair. a(2) – walk short distances.
B: desirability	b(1) – unable to help oneself. b(2) – would be able to do more activities.
C: prevention of movement	c(1) – people help me. c(2) – people ignore me.

The problem then becomes redefined as socially rather than mobility based. This would not mean necessarily abandoning the mobility plan but would demonstrate clearly that social reinforcement is more powerful than that of skill attainment. A new plan would be drafted giving the proper value to social needs.

Modelling

Bandura (1977) drew attention to the place which observation and modelling have in learning situations. This is discussed in the chapter on working with families. Clearly this is most likely to occur when the helper is valued and trusted. One of the most valued contributions a practitioner can make is to model a hopeful optimism which is rooted in reality and which does not discount a problem but demonstrated a creative ingenuity in tackling it. This is, of course, much easier to write than to achieve as are all the procedures described here.

Helper activities

To generate ideas in order to improve participation in the action plan the helper might include the following:

- Checking that the proposed incentives are effective.
- Checking that the programme is experienced as making a positive contribution to the life of the user or carer.
- Checking that the design of the programme is in keeping with the nature and demands of the tasks.
- Checking that the goal is seen to be of value by those people whose opinion matters to the user.

This list is by no means complete and no doubt helpers will be able to add ideas that they have found effective.

Programme monitoring

The way in which the programme will be monitored should be spelt out clearly at the beginning of the plan.

The purpose of *monitoring*, as its name suggests, is to warn the helper and the user of anything which may endanger the success of the planned problem management and alert them to adaptations which may need to be made.

The skills of *monitoring* are those which are used in both assessment and evaluation, as they are all part of the same process. They consist of observation and questioning. These may be incorporated into home visits, letters, telephone calls, questionnaires, reviews and case conferences. It is important that everyone is fully involved in the monitoring process and that the results are properly recorded.

The community practitioner has a number of roles. They are:

Coordinator
This involves ensuring that all the various contributions are dovetailing to provide adequate coverage of needs.

Quality controller
The practitioner is responsible for seeing that the services provided relate closely to the agreements reached. Changes should only occur in response to changes in need.

Supporter
The worker must be able to accept negative feedback, deal with it but not be overwhelmed by it. This positive outlook will ultimately provide the greatest support; it will aid service users, carers and other community practitioners.

Moderator
The practitioner will provide an overview of the whole helping process and make any necessary adjustments to the care plan, as the needs of users and carers change.

Recorder
The practitioner must keep a suitable record of the observations made and the result of other monitoring activities such as visiting and talking with service users, carers and other helpers. It will also provide material for supervision so the practitioner may also receive some supportive monitoring. Any changes made as a result of monitoring will also be recorded.

Evaluator

The worker will be assessing:

- the quality of participation of all concerned;
- the effectiveness of the objectives in maintaining movement towards the goal;
- the likely effectiveness of the goal in managing the problem situation;
- the nature of any changes that need to be made;
- the adequacy of the monitoring system in providing sufficient information, collected in a systematic way.

Participation in the monitoring process

Although the community practitioner has a responsibility to organise and record the monitoring process, his or her view of it is inevitably partial and incomplete.

Users and carers' contribution

These are vital if the records are to offer feedback on the success of the planned activity. This can be done by talking to those involved, but service users and carers can be encouraged to develop their own monitoring system and helped with its design, if this is required. Methods include:

- using time sheets to note *when* things happened;
- keeping diaries to record feelings/activities and experiences;
- devising activity checklists from which to monitor performances.

Other service providers

If a number of providers are involved, it is important that the monitoring procedures are known, shared and, if different, are accessible so that they can all contribute in the reviewing process.

That monitoring is sometimes neglected will come as no surprise after such a list of roles, all with a number of functions which are by no means straightforward. It is however absolutely essential if plans are to manage problems effectively. It should assist in the provision of a service which represents good value for money and prevents loss of motivation through faulty programme design.

The final evaluating stage

In some helping situations the level of need is such that, apart from necessary adjustments as circumstances change, some service input will always be required. In such cases the process is circular, requiring constant monitoring and review, leading to further planning, see scheme below.

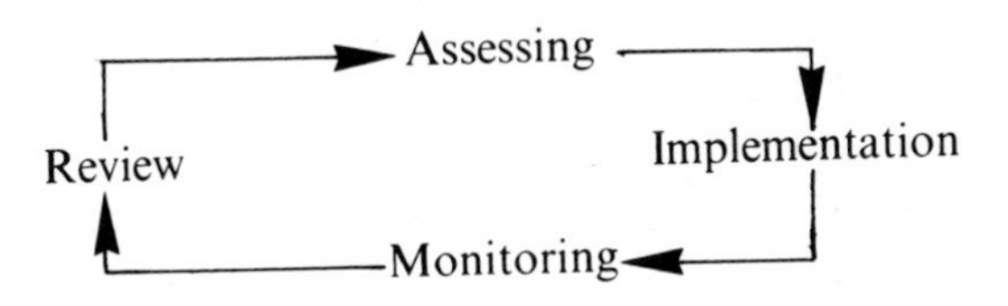

Even in these situations endings do occur and their management is particularly important when the dependency is of an ongoing nature. This section will look at:

1. Indicators which suggest when an ending may be appropriate.
2. The experience of ending, with particular focus on the user.
3. The tasks confronting the user and the helper at this stage.
4. Workers learning through the helping process.

Indicators that an ending may be appropriate

Some useful guidelines were developed by Maholick and Turner (1979). They were developed for a psychotherapeutic setting but are capable of much more general application. Factors included:

- degree of problem or symptom relief;
- the level of stress still experienced;
- the increase in coping ability;
- the increase in the valuing of self and others;
- increased levels of relating to others – of loving and being loved;
- increased ability to plan work productively;
- increased capacity to play and enjoy life.

The *procedures* through which these sort of perceptions will be arrived are the monitoring and reviewing which should be a standard part of any programme. They should be capable of determining whether or not the goals which have been reached have led to a successful management of the problem situation. This in turn will lead to the less concrete but nevertheless important concepts propounded by Maholick and Turner.

The *skills* are again those which are used in assessment and monitoring. They are based on observation and questioning techniques and employ similar methods of collecting feedback; mainly through interviews, questionnaires and observation schedules. Like any other evaluation process, they should be chosen in consultation with the other participants in the action plan, especially the user and/or carer. They will also be influenced by the needs of the agency and the procedural framework in which the practitioner operates.

The experience of ending

Exercise 6

Individually or in groups

Write down all the words which have associations with endings for you.

Think about what relevance these associations may have in your community practice.

You probably collected some positive and negative emotions connected with endings. Of course different endings have different meanings and arouse different feelings. Some reactions are present to a degree in many types of endings and will be briefly listed because they influence our work with people in this closing phase. (It is worth remembering that these endings are mutual and the community practitioner will also experience an emotional reaction as a working partnership draws to its close.)

Denial

There may be some fending off the reality of the end. 'I expect I shall still see you around' and similar responses. This will mean that the meaning of ending, when it is finally confronted, will be done alone. It helps later if there has been some shared acknowledgement of loss. It is important that practitioners do not collude with this denial because they too are finding the parting difficult.

Sadness

This may feel quite positive and often implies that the relationship has been valued and real, unless the grief is extreme. The ability to form a good working relationship can be taken forward into other situations and should be seen as a hopeful sign for future developments. Both practitioners and users will often share feelings of sadness at this time of ending.

Anger

Just as accepting help is not easy, neither will be the experience of its withdrawal. Some people will experience the ending as a minimisation of their needs. It is hard sometimes for both service user and community practitioners to accept the tight limits imposed upon them by resource restrictions. It may be possible to see valuable work that might be done if prioritisation was not such an issue. Practitioners also may feel angry because they have felt limited by the actions of the service users or the carers.

Appreciation
This is a good feeling for both helper and the person accepting help. It is the recognition that what has been received is good and this too may apply to both. It is a privilege to be allowed into the life of another person and is often an enriching experience for the practitioner as well as the service user.

Relief
Learning, as we have already noted, is stressful. Most useful interventions impose a level of stress and the prospect of its removal may seem quite welcome. This again is just as likely to be experienced by the community practitioner who may have experienced the whole relationship as a bit of an uphill slog.

The tasks of termination

The fact that endings tend to generate some quite strong emotions makes it particularly important that this stage of the relationship should be handled sensitively, respectfully and genuinely; the practitioner acknowledging that it is an end for them as well as for the other person or people involved. Important issues to consider at such times are:

The relationship between the worker and service user
The ups and downs of such a relationship may well be reviewed, not from self-indulgent nostalgia, but because it will contain learning which can be taken forward by everyone involved to improve the quality of their interactions.

The helping process
This will include an evaluation of each part of the 'helping process' – the assessment, the contract, the objectives, the goals, the implementation and the monitoring. These will be critically reviewed to see how far they were successful in diagnosing the difficulties, choosing goals which would contribute significantly to their management and adopting clear and workable objectives by which these goals may be reached. The implementation of plans and their

monitoring will also be evaluated to see whether they were capable of accommodating and responding to change.

This analysis will constitute important learning for the practitioner because it will enable him or her to identify deficits in both skills and resources which should be fed into the final written evaluation. They have important implications for supervision and training needs as well as for resource allocation and management.

The learning for the service users may include:

- an ability to identify areas which are stressful for them;
- an ability to discriminate more clearly between supportive and disabling environments;
- an ability to recognise their areas of strengths and a knowledge of how to exploit these in the management of their difficulties;
- the experience of having mastered problems which at first seemed unmanageable which can now be transferred into new relationships and situations.

Planning aftercare

Because of the demands of the final step it is important that the practitioner offers support not just in the review of the past and its implication for the future, but also by identifying in concrete ways what resources are available to the service user and how these may best be mobilised and used in the future. This will include consideration of resources within the family and immediate neighbourhood as well as the wider community. This may well include research into the existence and nature of resources as well as consideration of the most suitable method of referral, i.e. self referral or agency referral. The consideration given earlier to the referral process should be remembered here if the community practitioner is involved in the referral process.

How to say goodbye

Recognition of the ending should always be made when this is predictable. Of course there are no rules about how these endings should take place but it is an area of practice which is often neglected.

Exercise 7

Individually or in groups

1. Practitioners should consider whether their use of final sessions:

- Reflects the quality of the relationship.
- Reflects the quality of the work achieved.
- Values the achievements and strengths of the service users.

2. What difficulties do workers experience at this point?
3. How might these be dealt with more effectively?

The community practitioner's learning

A final evaluation checklist should include such questions as:

What have you learnt about yourself?
What have you learnt about your personal style of helping?
What have you learnt about the person/people with whom you worked?
What have you learnt about their world?
What have you learnt about your relationship with each other?
What have you learnt about your own helping agency?
What have you learnt about other helping agencies?
What have you learnt about the quality of resources available to this person?
What theoretical concepts have you used in arriving at these understandings?
What will this learning mean to you both personally and profesionally?

Implications for your agency

One of the reasons why detailed evaluation is important is that it can provide valuable feedback to your own agency.

Feedback on communication systems

These are usually tested during a sustained piece of work and any identification of where they are vulnerable should be noted and shared appropriately.

Feedback on information systems

Lack of information is often a problem for practitioners as well as clients. This may point to faults in the information system or may be the result of a lack of knowledge. Community practitioners may choose to be their own researchers, but if they are there should be an effective system for sharing this work to prevent duplication.

Feedback on resources

Practitioners will often be able to identify very accurately the strengths and weaknesses of the resources available and also those which are missing resulting in unmet needs. Clearly this is too important to remain the private or informal concern of individual practitioners.

Feedback on training and support
It is easy to blame onself when encountering difficulty. Sometimes, if the situation is analysed more carefully, it will be seen to be the result of a lack of training.

There are frequent changes in the demands on practitioners and continued training is essential if they are to adjust positively. Helpers need to be able to assert their needs for support and for training based on firm evidence from their current practice.

Conclusion

The community practitioner is in a difficult position, standing at the interface between the social service system and the individual's experience of difficulty. Of course there will be anger and disappointment as well as gratitude as the practitioner seeks to use the resources of the system to meet the needs of the individual. A planned and organised approach to the work should better equip the practitioner for what is a demanding, but rewarding, task.

References

Atherton, J. S. (1986) *Professional Supervision in Group Care, the Contract Based Approach*. London: Tavistock.

Bandura, A. (1977) *Social Learning Theory*. Englewood Cliffs, NJ: Prentice Hall.

Brechin, A. and Liddiard, P. (1981) *Look At It This Way – New Perspectives in Rehabilitation*. Milton Keynes: The Open University.

Charities Digest. Published annually by The Family Welfare Association.

Egan, G. (1990) The Skilled Helper – a Systematic Approach to Effective Helping. California: Brooks/Cole.

Herbert, M. (1985) *Caring for you Children: a Practical Guide*. Oxford: Basil Blackwell.

King's Fund Library. The King's Fund Centre, 126 Albert Street, London NW1 7NF.

Mager, R. F. (1974) *Goal Analysis*. California: Pitman Learning.

Maholick, L. T. and Turner, D. W. (1979) Termination: that difficult farewell. *American Journal of Psychotherapy*, **33,** 583–592.

National Children's Bureau: 8 Wakley Street, London EC1V 7QE.

Priestly, P., McGuire, J., Flegg, D., Hemsley V. and Welham, D. (1978) *Social Skills and Personal Problem Solving – a Handbook of Methods*. London: Tavistock.

Seligman, M. E. P. (1975) *Helplessness: on Depression, Development and Death*. San Francisco: W. H. Freeman.

Tschudi, F. (1977) Loaded and honest questions: a construct theory view of symptoms and therapy. In Bannister, D. (ed) *New Perspectives in Personal Construct Theory*. London: Academic Press.

Chapter 8

Working with families

Val Jones

Introduction

Much community-based work is carried out with individuals. It might be argued that this is the only practical approach since it is individuals who suffer illnesses or accidents or who have disabilities, and it is individuals therefore who require some form of professional intervention. This perspective, whilst offering a simple and convenient framework for intervention, does overlook the known effects of a range of factors external to the individual in both the causation and outcome of many conditions. Environmental conditions – physical, social and emotional – are widely accepted as relevant considerations. Physical conditions are relatively easy to identify if not change; the social and emotional context of a person's life is much more difficult to come to grips with, for a variety of reasons.

The traditional model which regards illness as residing solely in the person influences professionals and lay people alike, so there is a shared expectation that the focus of professional activity will be the individual. Most community-based practitioners are trained and feel equipped to assess the needs of one person, to carry out a planned piece of work and evaluate the result. The assessment of a family or community network may appear to lie outside the practitioner's remit, or, even if accepted as important, seem too complex a task to tackle. In addition, practitioner self protection, an important consideration in a situation of limited resources and seemingly unlimited demand, should not be overlooked. Murgatroyd and Woolfe (1985) comment,

> Burn out is reduced when the helper feels most in control of a situation and for many this occurs when the relationship he or she has with a 'client' is on a one to one basis (p. 4).

So the 'medical model', coupled with practitioners' own need to manage and control their workload and avoid excessive stress, encourages an emphasis on individual needs assessment and intervention, even where it is clear to the practitioner that family and social factors are important and that a more family-focused approach could be helpful. This chapter seeks to offer a framework for understanding what the influence of families and other networks may be and how they create their effect. It suggests ways in which practitioners, without becoming specialist family practitioners, may become more skilled in managing family situations to the benefit of all concerned, particularly the identified client.

Family influences from the past

Whether a person is currently part of a family group or not, their family experiences will be significant.

> The family has an enduring impact on the development of the person. The family shapes the child's personality, attitudes, behaviour and beliefs. Although a person may change in some respects during his [*sic*] lifetime, the influence of the family . . . cannot be completely undone. (Thorman 1982, p. 1)

Children learn from their parents in a variety of ways, some of which are intended and some not. All parents make conscious efforts, usually by means of reward and punishment, to inculcate in their children 'acceptable' behaviour and values; what is acceptable is determined partially by social factors such as class and partially by factors unique to the family concerned. In addition, children model themselves on their parents or caretakers in quite unconscious ways, as any parent who has been embarrassed to observe their words and non-verbal behaviour faithfully reproduced by toddlers will testify. Attitudes and behaviour learned at this very early stage, may remain powerful in adulthood, and again those who find themselves repeating much disliked parental admonitions to their own children may find this unsurprising.

A brief exploration of the nature of attitudes may help clarify why childhood learning remains so influential. Bem (1970, p. 14) offers one of the simplest definitions of attitudes, 'attitudes are likes and dislikes'. However, it is generally assumed by social psychologists that the positive or negative feeling component of attitudes (likes and dislikes) is supported by a set of beliefs and that, other things being equal, there is a tendency to behave in a way consistent with those feelings and beliefs. Children absorb the feeling and behavioural aspects of parental attitudes long before they are able to understand the underlying beliefs. In other words, the attitude is already in place before the reason for it is understood. Hence the 7-year-old who could say, 'I don't know any black people and I don't want to, thank you' (7 Up, Granada TV, 1963). It might be supposed though that as they grow up and are subjected to other influences and information people's attitudes will change and this is to some extent true. Human beings do not however always respond on the basis of reason. Rather, new information is filtered through existing attitudes and beliefs, and where it conflicts with them may be rejected or compartmentalised. Even where it is accepted, there is a period of psychological discomfort or dissonance while it is assimilated, especially if a change of attitude is required. In other words, information will not necessarily influence attitudes, so early learning is not easily undone. A concrete example concerning attitudes to illness may help to illustrate the point. For those who are interested in discovering more about attitude formation, further reading is suggested at the end of the chapter.

Consider for a moment how illness was regarded in the family you grew up in. How was 'illness' defined? How ill did you have to be not to go to school, for instance? How were you treated when ill? What feelings did illness generate in your family? Was it more acceptable for some members of the family to be ill than others? How were doctors and other health professionals regarded? Now consider your current attitude to illness in yourself or other members of your family. It would be surprising if this did not reflect some of your earlier experiences.

Helpers may argue, however, that their view of illness or handicap in their professional role differs from their personal approach. It is at least possible that those clients whose attitude to their condition corresponds more closely to the practitioners' own are more satisfying to work with than those who have a very different one. In fact, since many of those who choose to be helpers tend to minimise their own ailments, I would venture to suggest that the client who shows a determination to overcome difficulties is viewed in a more positive light than the one who seems rather passive or even reluctant to get well.

This is but one example of how values and attitudes learned in the family may exert an often unconscious influence on current behaviour. Standards of cleanliness and hygiene, expectations of men and women, especially as husbands and fathers or wives and mothers, approaches to money management, child rearing practices, attitudes to outsiders', especially professionals, are among the many others.

Exercise

Select a person with whom you are working or have recently worked and with whom you feel you have had a positive and productive relationship

- Consider their attitude to their illness or condition.
- Consider their attitude to you as a professional.
- Identify any other factors about the person and their values which you think may have contributed to the successful relationship.
- Repeat the exercise in relation to a person with whom you feel you have had a less productive working relationship.

Was it the case that the first person was either more similar to you or more nearly met your expectations of how a person of that gender or age should behave? Whether or not this was so, a degree of scepticism may remain about just how far people are victims of their upbringing. There can be little doubt in the minds of community-based practitioners about the significance of the family when the client is part of an existing family group. The power of other family members to influence outcomes for good or ill is apparent and in the latter case a family focus may be useful.

What is a family?

Most people have experience of family life since the family, however defined, is the basic social unit in most societies. There have also been many attempts at formal definitions, some of which are discussed in Chapter 3. Ultimately each person's understanding of the family is an amalgam of personal experience and knowledge gained from other sources. The approach taken here is one which has become increasingly popular in the psychosocial helping professions such as psychiatry and social work in the past few decades as a basis for intervening in family situations; that is the systems approach.

The simple premise at the heart of systems theory is that the whole is greater than the sum of its parts, and that a study of the parts in isolation from each other will not sufficiently explain the relationships between them which give rise to the whole. In the case of a mechanical system, such as a watch, careful examination of the constituent parts will give an understanding of each component and its attributes, but not of the interaction between them, though it is that which turns them from a heap of bits into a functioning timepiece.

If this is translated into human terms, and applied to the family, then the components are the family members and the attributes their personal characteristics. The family functions and carries out its socially allotted tasks by means of the communications, both verbal and non-verbal, which go on between those members. Each person, like each watch part, contributes uniquely to the system but is also affected by their relationship with the other members.

The focus is upon interaction and the effects one person may have on another rather than upon any innate qualities of the individuals involved. For example, mothers of children with disabilities may be described by professionals as 'over-protective' (an innate characteristic). It might equally be said that the child is 'lazy' or 'unwilling to help him- or herself', though this is much more unlikely! From a systems perspective, it is the relationship between the two which is important and how each influences the other to behave in particular ways. This idea will be developed later in the chapter, but first a little more theoretical background might be useful.

The family as a system

The family, when viewed as a system, is seen to have certain features which it is necessary for practitioners to understand. These have been usefully summarised by a number of writers (e.g. Manor 1984; Bennun 1988). The key characteristics are listed below.

1. The family as a system is self-aware, that is the family members know who is within the family and who is not.
2. Each family system contains sub-systems, e.g. the marital and parental pair, the children, a close mother–son or father–daughter pair.
3. Each family system operates within a social environment or supra-system made up of extended family, neighbourhood, and other systems such as church, school or hospital.
4. The family system has a boundary which is recognised by those inside and outside the family. Families may be closed systems, having a clearly defined boundary and minimal contact with the outside world, or open systems in which there is a great deal of interaction between family members and other people and organisations.
5. Within the family, too, there may be boundaries between sub-systems which will affect communication between family members.

6. The family needs to both maintain itself as a functioning system carrying out basic tasks (usually the provision of food, shelter and care to its members) and to respond to demands for change either from within the family, e.g. the birth of a new baby, or from the environment, e.g. a child reaching school age.

A good starting point for testing these ideas is to look at one's own family. The exercise which follows is designed to help focus in a more concrete way on some of the features of family systems outlined above.

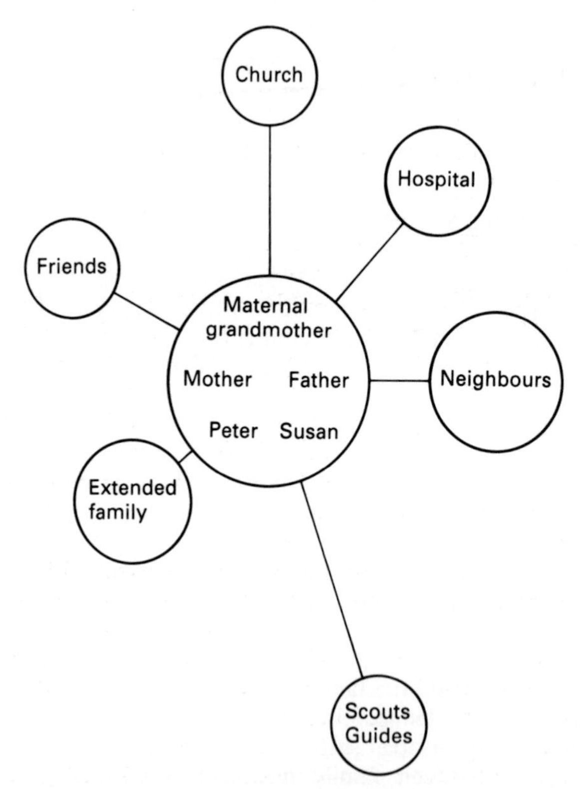
Church
Hospital
Friends
Maternal grandmother
Mother
Father
Peter
Susan
Neighbours
Extended family
Scouts Guides
How much or how little these impinge upon the family can be illustrated by their closeness to or distance from the centre. Each family's supra system will be slightly different.

Figure 8.1 The family

Exercise

- Draw a large circle and write or draw within it all whom you regard as belonging to your family (Figure 8.1) (if easier, take your family of origin at some point in the past) (see 1, p. 213).
- Draw dotted circles around any sub-systems which you think exist or existed (N.B. these may overlap since family members may be part of a number of sub-systems) (see 2, p. 213).
- Around the outside of the circle indicate important aspects of the social environment or supra-system (see 3, p. 213).
- Consider the boundary between the family and the outside world. How much contact do or did the family have with outsiders, either informally in the shape of friends and neighbours or formally through membership of organisations? (see 4, p. 213).

If it is possible to share the outcome of this exercise with others who have completed it differences will be apparent. There is no blueprint for the perfect family. Class, culture, race and the family experiences and expectations brought by each partner into a new relationship will affect all aspects of family life.

Families vary both in their capacity to carry out the basic tasks and to cope with demands placed upon them from within and without. These variations are related to a family's ability to accommodate the progressive stages of the family life cycle, the nature of the basic processes which maintain the system and the quality of the social environment in which the family operates (Thorman 1982). Each of these will be considered in turn.

The family life-cycle

Regardless of social context, each family, like each individual, has to negotiate a series of developmental stages. These stages are of course closely linked to individual growth and development. The family life-cycle 'can be seen as a sequence of characteristic stages beginning with the formation of the family through to its dissolution' (Bennun 1988, p. 15).

A number of writers (e.g. Hughes *et al.* 1978; Carter and McGoldrick 1980) have offered models of the family life-cycle. The one used here is based on that of Hughes *et al.*

- Beginning families include courtship, marriage and the period prior to the birth of the first child.

- Child-bearing families start when the first child is born.
- Child-rearing families are a continuation of the previous stage, when the children in the family are pre-adolescent.
- Families with teenagers start when the first child reaches puberty.
- Families as launching centres span the period of time during which the children are leaving home.
- Families in the middle years cover the time when parents are alone after the departure of the children and before retirement.
- Ageing families encompass the years from retirement to death.

Each of these developmental stages requires adjustments on the part of family members if they are to be negotiated successfully and families, as already indicated, find the transitions more or less difficult. For example, the advent of a first child, however much wanted, offers a challenge to the pattern of life which has been established by a couple. Few couples find it possible to continue in the same way as before, though this may be their hope and expressed intention prior to the birth! This wish for sameness, sometimes referred to as the system's drive towards homeostasis (a steady state), produces tension when the need for change becomes pressing. At the other end of the spectrum, the responsibility of caring for an elderly, ailing parent, however much loved, has a similar effect.

Before considering how families manage to maintain themselves and to develop, a brief word of caution about the life-cycle model is in order. Although it is clear that every family has developmental changes to cope with, the neat two-parent, two-point-four child, white middle class nuclear family is not the only one. Childless couples, three-generational families, reconstituted families, homosexual and lesbian pairings, whether these include children or not, and many other variations on the theme of family life are important too. The model is just that, rather than a prescription for normality. However, the framework does have value for a practitioner confronted with a difficult family situation, as will be illustrated below.

Family roles and relationships

When two people embark upon a long-term relationship – and for the sake of simplicity let us assume it is a marriage – they enter uncharted waters. Each is taking on a new role, as husband or wife, and their expectations of what those roles will involve have already been formed to some degree by both general socialisation and experiences in their family of origin. Who will manage the money?

Who will do the cooking? the cleaning? the decorating? All these are areas for negotiation, much of which will take place at an implicit rather than explicit level, only emerging when serious disagreement occurs.

Each partner has views not only about their own role but about the other too. A cautionary tale from an erstwhile colleague concerned a coke boiler. In the early days of her marriage the coke boiler frequently went out and was the subject of mutual recriminations. In her family, her father always dealt with the fires, whereas in her husband's his mother did. Each thus saw it as the other's responsibility. The purchase of oil-fired central heating averted divorce but the point seemed well made. I am sure readers can provide their own examples.

As the relationship develops and if children appear, the roles of mother and father are added, and another, equally powerful, set of expectations comes into operation, not just about parental roles but about how children should behave. The demands of the life-cycle continue to require change and development not just of the couple but of surrounding family members. For every newly married couple there are two couples coping with 'in-law' status, and for every parent two grandparents. So, if the system is to maintain itself and change, a constant, if often unobtrusive, process of role negotiation is called for.

Another key issue for any couple to deal with is that of intimacy versus separateness or autonomy. For a relationship to remain in existence, each person must get enough out of it to make it better than being alone. We all have varying needs for personal space and for closeness, and varying ways of expressing those needs. Some families are very physical, with lots of kisses and cuddles, others do not go in for overt emotional displays. Some families 'do everything together', in others individuals follow their own hobbies and interests with little reference to each other. As long as everyone is happy, it is not important. However, it is unlikely that either needs or experiences will be perfectly matched, so it is another arena for negotiation. Which is to say that it, like role, is a potential source of conflict which the system has to contend with.

A few concrete examples may help to underline the point, which is really about the (largely unspoken) 'rules' of the relationship. Is it all right for one or other partner to go out alone? bring a friend home unexpectedly? spend money without consultation? Who initiates sexual activity? Where and when does sex happen? These and many other questions are addressed and resolved, usually without either person being aware that such a thing has occurred. The birth of a child means that three new relationships must be developed and maintained, i.e. mother/baby; father/baby; mother/father. The old husband–wife relationship will also need reworking. Even if children are never part of the scene, there will be changes as the relationship matures.

It is often easier to be aware of the roles and relationship rules in families other than our own. Generally, such things only become apparent when the rules are broken or a family member takes over a task normally owned by someone else.

Exercise
Consider your own family or one you know well (not necessarily one with whom you are working).

- Are roles very clearly defined or rather flexible?
- Can you identify any relationship rules?
- Are there different rules for different family members?
- What seems to affect these? age? gender? other factors such as pressure from extended family?
- Can you identify any points of change in roles or relationships related to the changing life-cycle?
- If possible, compare your findings with others who have completed the exercise. It is easy to assume that our own experience is 'normal' and use it as a blueprint for others' family life even though we know that families vary.

Families and major change

What have been described above are the normal processes of change and adjustment occurring over the life of a family. These are sometimes referred to in the literature as 'first order changes'. However, most families will also have to cope at some time with more dramatic or 'second order change'. Second order change, which has been described as 'the difference that makes a difference', challenges the family system much more fundamentally.

The birth of a child is a first order change; the birth of a handicapped child can be seen as a second order change since normal expectations have to be suddenly re-evaluated. Other examples might be the unexpected incapacitation of the breadwinner by an accident; divorce or separation; the death of a child (as opposed to the death of an elderly person, which, although distressing, is expected in the normal course of events); unemployment or major external events like war. All of these call into question a family's established ways of coping and demand major adjustments. Possible responses in such crisis situations will be considered below.

Family interaction patterns

In the earlier discussion, there has been a good deal of emphasis placed upon negotiation and little upon conflict though the former implies the possibility of the latter. In fact, all family systems have to find ways of coping with the inevitable conflicts that arise over both trivial and more serious matters in the best regulated households. How well conflicts around roles, relationships and any other issues are dealt with depends to a considerable extent upon the communication patterns which have evolved.

The key to understanding families from the systems perspective is through the interaction of family members. Minuchin (1974) says,

> A family is a system which operates through transactional patterns. Repeated transactions establish patterns of how, when, and to whom to relate and these patterns underpin the system.

Communication in families, as in other human situations, takes place at a number of levels. There are clear, explicit verbal messages which mean what they say ('I'm very happy that you've been successful'); there are verbal messages which are confused and confusing ('Of course I don't mind what you do – as long as you don't cause me any worry'); there are verbal messages which are clearly in conflict with the accompanying non-verbal behaviour ('Yes, it's fine for you to go out for a drink' – while the noise level involved in washing up increases ten-fold); finally there is silence, either comfortable or of the variety which speaks volumes (Murgatroyd and Woolfe 1985).

In an ideal world all communication would be of the open, straightforward kind, a vehicle for the sharing of information and feelings, for seeking help when needed, for offering support to others. Unfortunately, life is rarely perfect and, whilst most families have 'good enough' communication, patterns evolve which may inhibit the development of individual members and/or the whole family. The complexity of family communication is such that it is only possible to touch on some of the aspects which may be of particular interest to community practitioners.

At a family meal the conversation flowed but it was noticeable that whenever the middle daughter (aged about 11) was asked a question her mother answered for her. This pattern had probably started many years before when the child had hearing problems but once established had continued. The same child was often described as 'not listening'. This is a simple example of a fairly harmless pattern; others can be more complex and more destructive.

At bedtime, father asked his elder son to go to bed and began to get irritable when he did not respond immediately. The younger son demanded attention and his father turned on him crossly. At this point mother intervened, accusing her husband of unfairly picking on the younger son. The parents' argument developed, and the elder son tried to smooth things over. Father redirected his anger to the boy; his younger brother started to jump around noisily, distracting father, who again started to admonish him. Mother accused father . . . and the whole situation escalated, night after night. These parents eventually sought help because of their difficulty in controlling the children.

It would be easy, in the above situation, to 'blame' one or other members of the family. A case could be made for each one being responsible: the older boy for refusing to go to bed in the first place, his brother for interfering, father for being short-tempered and unfair or mother for criticising her husband for favouring the younger son. The systemic perspective focuses upon the circular nature of the interaction, which follows 'rules', unrecognised by the family concerned but very powerful none the less.

Virginia Satir (1972) has identified four common 'roles' in families where communication is difficult. These are: Blamer, Placator, Distractor and Computer. Computer is used to describe a person who shows no emotion and offers an apparently rational perspective at all times. Blamer, of course, holds other people responsible for everything that happens, Placator tries to smooth things over and Distractor creates a diversion, by either saying or doing something quite irrelevant to the subject under discussion.

Exercise

If you are able to find two or three other people to work with, form yourselves into a 'family group'. Choose roles (as above) and set yourselves the task of discussing, for example, the next family holiday or arrangements for Christmas. After 5 minutes or so review how the discussion has gone, and how people feel in their role. It is sometimes possible to recognise faint traces of oneself in one or other of the roles and the discussion is unlikely to have reached a conclusion.

This exercise underlines the concept of circular rather than linear causation. It is usually difficult to single out one person as the one responsible for the problems, though it is likely that everyone involved feels that it was the others who sabotaged the discussion.

Practitioners are often puzzled that although families say very clearly that they want to change, long and earnest discussions result in little or no movement. The mother of two teenage children who were playing a game and kept asking for help remarked, 'I hoped that by now you would be able to play on your own'. As she spoke, she joined them on the floor and began to help both. The expressed wish for change was contradicted by her actions, which is not to suggest that it was not a genuine wish. The message for practitioners is that what families do is a much more important indicator than what they say.

It is a central tenet of systems theory that whatever is going on in a family is a form of communication and that it serves some purpose, otherwise it would imply fade away. Even behaviour patterns which are causing obvious discomfort to one or more people cannot be dismissed. In fact, it is likely that they are important and may well represent the family's attempt to avoid conflict and stay together. Oded Manor (1984) suggests looking for the 'positive value of apparently distressing behaviour' as a starting point for intervention.

A family was brought to the attention of the hospital social work department because of the number of admissions the 5-year-old had had with severe asthma attacks. On investigation, it was discovered that the parents' relationship was very unsatisfactory and that father had actually moved out. However, whenever the child was admitted to hospital both parents came together over his bed. He had taken the responsibility for keeping them together, at serious risk to his own health. Work with the parents on their relationship, aimed at helping them to confront their differences, resulted in a dramatic drop in the number and severity of the attacks.

The child, in this instance, was the 'symptom carrier' for the family. In a similar way the over-protected child mentioned earlier may well not help himself because the family depends upon him to maintain the status quo, and he knows that any change might rock the boat. In some families a scapegoat is found who literally carries all the difficulties, and allows other family members to feel that they are all right. It cannot be over emphasised that, in these examples, the participants are not aware of the process, though it may be very clear to an outsider, especially one who thinks in a systemic way.

Exercise

Think of a family with whom you are involved where what the family *says* it wants is, for example, for the identified client to 'get better', 'become more independent', but where, despite your best efforts, no change apparently occurs. Consider what the benefits of the current situation might be for individuals and for the maintenance of the system, and what their fears might be about change. Take the opportunity to speculate about possibilities.

The last aspect of family communication addressed here concerns alliances, coalitions and hierarchy. All these processes assume at least three members in the family. We have discussed earlier the existence of sub-systems and it sometimes happens that two or more people form an alliance. Alliances are positive in that the two may unite to share a hobby or plan a treat for other family members. Coalitions, on the other hand, tend to be set up for the purpose of attacking or undermining another member of the family. Common examples would be a coalition between a grandparent and grandchild which undermines the authority of the parents, or between a father and daughter which excludes the mother. Coalitions can exert a powerful influence upon patterns of interaction.

Hierarchy is concerned with the distribution of executive power in the family, that is who makes the decisions. Cross-generational coalitions such as those suggested above may control the communication and decision-making processes. It is essential for practitioners to be aware of such possibilities since, for work to be effective, the powerful people must be recognised.

Family communication is a fascinating topic and one which repays more investigation than has been possible here. It, like other aspects of family life, is influenced by the context in which it occurs.

The suprasystem

There is a danger of accepting the systemic approach, but limiting it to the family so that blame is shifted from the individual to the family, overlooking the effect of the environment on that family's functioning. For some the extended family, neighbourhood and community are benign and supportive, for others hostile and even dangerous. Poverty, poor housing, racism and other social phenomena may affect internal dynamics as well as the relationship between the family and the outside world. Experience of these as well as of agencies such as the Health Service and Social Services may drive families to ways of coping which are then seen as dysfunctional by professionals. It may also put them in conflict with each other and the services concerned.

This brief overview of some of the ideas underlying the systems perspective is intended only to stimulate thinking and to challenge the purely individual approach. The concluding exercise offers an opportunity to put together these ideas in relation to work before moving on to look at practical applications.

Exercise

(a) Choose a family with whom you are working, or have worked, and which has experienced sudden illness, accident or deterioration in one member.
(b) Describe the condition of the person identified as the client, including any implications that might have for example for their everyday functioning.
(c) Consider how this change has affected all family members in terms of:

- family roles;
- relationships within the family;
- communication patterns;
- relationships with the outside world.

(d) What are the needs of individuals and the needs of the family as a whole? (There may be conflicts here.)
(e) What impact do you feel (c) and (d) are having upon your capacity to help?

Some practical techniques

This concluding section offers some practical ideas for understanding and working with families based on the systemic approach. The practitioner needs to be able to build up a picture of the family, to observe interaction in an unbiased way and to hypothesise about what may be happening. Thus it is helpful to see as many of the close family members as possible, at least on an initial visit. This issue will be discussed further when considering the last and crucial issue of communicating with families.

Building up a picture

Everyone is familiar with the idea of a family tree or genogram but its use as a way to 'gather, organise and store information' when working with a family may be less well known. The traditional social history usually takes the form of a list of family members and a written account of background information. This does not help the practitioner to see the family relationships clearly, whereas the genogram can 'provide an overall view of complex family constellations in an extremely concise and efficient form' (Burnham 1990, p. 27).

There are certain recognised symbols used by family therapists and these are shown in Figure 8.2, but it can also be used

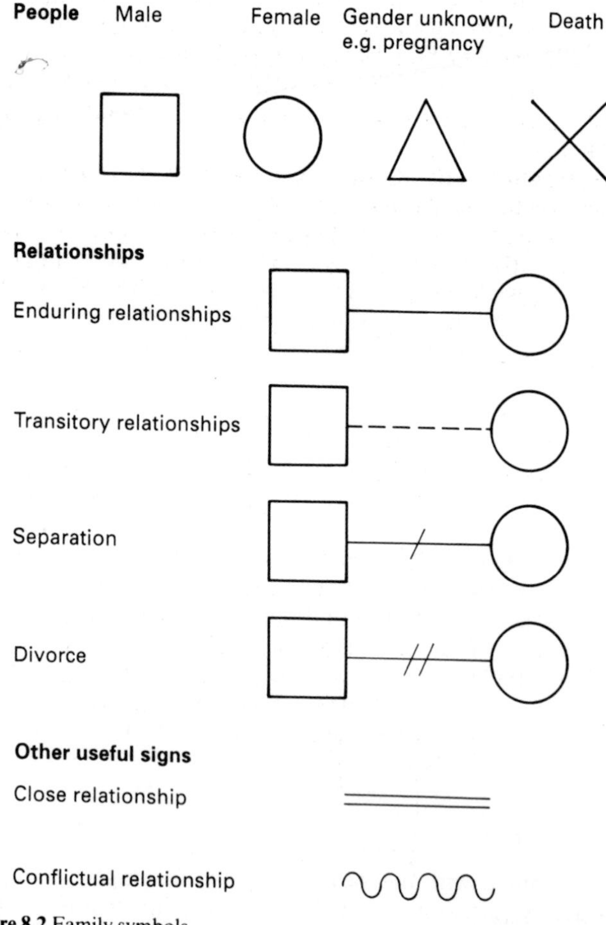

Figure 8.2 Family symbols

individually and creatively to record information beyond the basic data. Burnham suggests that a complete genogram should include: names and ages of all family members; exact dates of birth, marriage, separation, divorce, death and other significant life events; notations with dates about occupation, places of residence, illness and other changes in life course; information on three or more generations. Genograms are often completed in conjunction with the family but this is not essential, especially where the primary task is not family work. Figure 8.2 outlines the basic symbols used.

For example, a genogram for the family with the asthmatic child might look like that shown in Figure 8.3.

If the family is a reconstituted one, the relationship can become very complicated and that is reflected better in visual than in written form. Genograms do not necessarily have to be limited to family members; other significant relationships with friends, neighbours or even other professionals can also be included. It is a tool that can be developed by helpers to suit their own needs and particular situations.

Another technique which may help a practitioner to come to grips with family relationships and interaction is sculpting. This technique is often used directly with families, when a family member is asked by the worker to arrange their family as they see them and/or as they would wish them to be. A series of sculpts, directed by

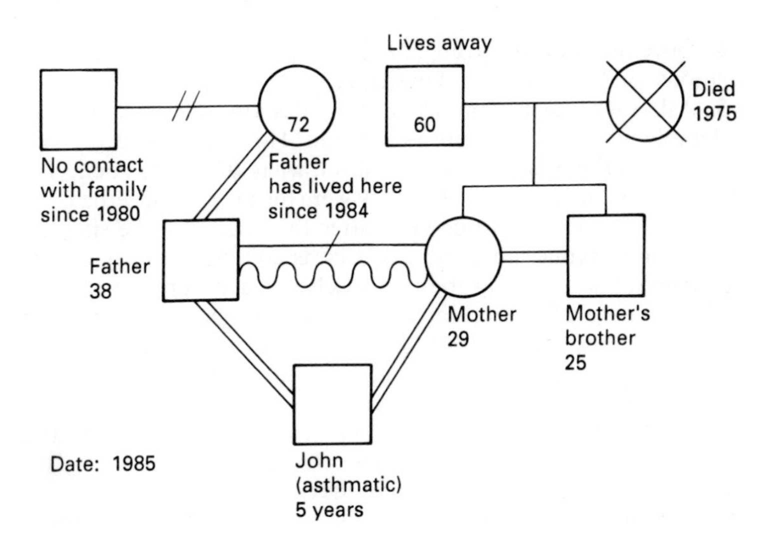

Figure 8.3 Family genogram

different people, can give a range of perspectives. That is not what is being suggested here. Rather it is offered as an action-based approach to understanding the experiences of various family members.

A sculpt has some similarities to a role play in that it is an exercise in empathic imagination, but it involves neither speech nor movement. It is a 'snapshot' of a family as seen by one person, in this case the practitioner, who needs to direct the sculpt. Its value is in hearing from the participants how they felt during the process.

Setting up a sculpt

1. Gather together a willing group of friends or colleagues, sufficient to represent the family members (these may include members whom the practitioner has not met but whom the family has spoken of and who seem to be important).

2. There is no need to give the participants any information about the family. In fact the less information they have the better.

3. Allocate roles and arrange the participants as you see the family. How close are the various people to each other? Are they touching or a long way apart? Who is looking at whom? Are some members looking away? What kinds of gestures are being made – loving, supplicatory, rejecting, indifferent? What about facial expressions? Is one or more members dominant, needing to be placed higher up, or submissive?

It is best for the director to do the arranging physically as far as possible.

4. Once the sculpt is arranged, ask the participants to hold their positions for 30 seconds or so in silence.

5. Ask each participant in turn to describe their experience, preferably whilst they remain in position. How do they feel? What are the good things about their position, what are not so good? Try to encourage them to speak as if they were the person concerned.

6. It is a good idea to de-brief after this exercise. The simplest way is for everyone, once the feedback is complete, to say clearly their name and something about themselves, e.g. occupation.

The purpose of the sculpt is to give the practitioner another perspective. Experience suggests that hearing the feedback can broaden the practitioner's view and offer alternative ways of dealing with situations. One of its particular values may be in hearing how a person labelled as 'the problem', perhaps that over-protective mother or bossy husband, is feeling. Despite its artificiality, the sculpt may present another aspect of the truth.

A perhaps extreme example is of a sculpt in which the 3-year-old daughter, whom it was felt was being rejected by the family, was actually left out by the practitioner/director. In this case, the message about the strength of what the family was conveying was underlined, focusing attention on the need to take it, and the risk to the child, seriously.

A sculpt can also be a useful tool to look at other systems, for example a work team, and identify what is going on there. A not uncommon phenomenon in staff teams is that of scapegoating and to do this exercise, either with the team or with substitutes, can clarify what is happening and help understanding.

Observation

It is essential that a practitioner who regards interaction as important should be able to observe, in as unbiased a way as possible. We have seen earlier that one of the major blocks is likely to be our own family experience which colours interpretation of what is going on in others. A person who comes from a family where rows are rare and, when they occur, are serious, is at risk of misconstruing their significance in a family which conducts most of its affairs in an adversarial but friendly way!

In order to minimise bias, it is helpful to have some kind of yardstick against which to observe. Several authors provide observation checklists of this kind and two of these are reproduced here.

Thorman (1982) offers the following list of questions for practitioners to ask themselves about family communication.

- Are family members able to be honest with each other about factual matters and about positive and negative feeling? Can people admit problems to each other and be open about what they want from each other?
- How skilled are family members at listening to each other?
- How do family members negotiate about things and decide on rules? Can they compromise?
- How are family responsibilities shared out?
- Do family members demonstrate positive feelings for each other verbally and non-verbally? Do they have fun together?
- How are individual differences and growth needs catered for? Are appropriate limits set?
- Is the family characterised by excessive amounts of: evasions and denials; double meanings; answering and speaking for others; giving orders; placating; blaming; sarcastic comments; inappropriate jokes; interruptions; put downs; bribes; defiance and rule breaking?

- Is there evidence of: collusions; scapegoating; hidden agendas (related to unspoken needs, wishes, emotional conflicts); secrets; myths or taboos; power struggles; lack of or too rigid boundaries.

This list covers most of the aspects of family communication mentioned earlier in the chapter and can help in making sense of what may be a confusing situation.

Manor (1984) has a similar checklist, but he divides his into three sections – communication, atmosphere and boundaries – which are the areas practitioners need to be aware of when observing a family group. What follows is a slightly simplified version of Manor's format.

1. Communication

- Notice pathways of communication:
  - eye contact between members
  - the direction of gestures
  - the movement of people in the group
  - who talks to whom?
  - who talks for whom?
- Notice the clarity of the communication.
- Notice the congruence between verbal and non-verbal messages.
- What is the frequency and type of control messages?
- How does the family deal with conflicts, expressions of feeling etc?
- Who initiates the discussion of what topic? Who responds, who is left out, who distracts attention from the topic?

2. Atmosphere

- Notice the mood of family members when together.
- Notice the mood of individual members.
  - How well are differences between members recognised?
- What is the tone of communications?
  - does the family show affection and appreciation?
  - is behaviour largely attacking or argumentative?
  - what range of feelings is expressed?
- Is humour part of the family experience?
- What sort of laughter is heard?

3. Boundaries

- How clear are the roles in the family?
  - parent/child
  - husband/wife
  - grandparent/parent
- How appropriate are the roles for the family's life stage?
- What are the coalitions in the family?

The last section (boundaries) can be particularly relevant to working with a family where one member is ill or disabled. Parents of children who have a disability (either physical or mental) may find it difficult to allow them to develop through the normal stages and the family may become 'stuck' at the 'child-rearing stage' even when the person is adult. Equally, if an adult child becomes disabled the family may revert to an earlier life stage. The relative rigidity of roles is also important in adjusting to change demanded by serious illness. If the practitioner can be sensitive to these matters, it is easier for both parties, since expectations can be modified on the one side, and threat reduced on the other. There is also the possibility of discussing the difficulty openly, once it has been recognised.

Hypothesising

This section will be brief, since it is largely a reminder of the importance of recognising the positive value of apparently distressing behaviour. When confronted with behaviour which seems destructive or self-defeating to an outsider it is useful to hypothesise about the meaning of such behaviour. However, such hypotheses are not necessarily correct and need to be constantly re-evaluated in the light of continuing work.

Another fruitful area for hypothesis concerns the transitions which may have triggered damaging patterns. The genogram is useful here. When data about the family are assembled in that form, major changes such as unemployment, emigration, accident or death are seen clearly. This can provide at the least an opportunity for discussion of how they may have affected family relationships. The same caution applies to these hypotheses, of course.

Communicating with families

The first question for the practitioner is, 'Who is the family?' and the second, 'How many of them do I need to see?'. Both of these are difficult to answer and are much discussed in the literature. Often, practitioners see only a small part of the family, although others may be present in spirit and feel quite powerful. A degree of assertiveness is required to ask to meet these absentees, but the discussion of a treatment or of a particular problem can offer an opportunity to suggest a family conference.

The importance of 'seeing for yourself' is that otherwise only one view of the system is available. It is easy, when working with an individual who is describing their partner, parent or child in the most negative terms either to accept their view without question, or, alternatively, to feel intensely sorry for the other person. In both cases, the effect is the same; the practitioner is drawn into the system and ceases to be able to observe what is happening or to help as effectively.

Although it may sound daunting, a discussion where family members speak for themselves rather than being reported at second-hand, and feelings are aired, can be very economical of time in the long run. It may have the effect of making people feel valued and important and therefore more committed to helping. Of course, it may also highlight the strength of feeling and disagreement, but at least that enables the practitioner to make an informed decision about the value of continuing work!

Once the family members have been assembled, it is helpful for the practitioner to have a framework for managing the situation. One of the pioneers of family therapy, Jay Haley (1974), drew up a comprehensive description of the initial interview and his model has been adapted here.

Interviewing

An interview with a family involves four stages:

- the social stage
- the problem stage
- the interaction stage
- the definition of change.

The social stage involves meeting with everyone and engaging them. It is important to speak personally to each person present and if possible to have some exchange with them, about the weather, journey etc. This stage also provides an opportunity for the practitioner to begin to observe relationships and roles.

The problem stage is a time for finding out what each person present sees as the difficulty, if there is one. If the purpose of the meeting is to discuss plans rather than address a particular problem then each person's view of the current situation would be valuable. Again, it is important to try and speak with each person, but this may prove hard to do, depending on the family pattern of communication. Often it is most difficult to get a view from the person most directly concerned, especially if that happens to be someone who is disabled or old. Continuing observation of the family communication at this stage, and the following one will help the practitioner develop understanding of the family dynamics.

The interaction stage is an opportunity for the family to talk the problem or the situation through, since it is the family who will be responsible for managing in the long term. If the practitioner can take a back seat and allow this discussion to develop, that is good. Families, though, often see the practitioner as the expert and persist in addressing remarks 'through the chair'. As far as possible try to redirect these comments, thus underlining the central role of the family.

Change definition, the concluding part of the interview, is about deciding upon goals for the future. If the family can reach agreement on desired and attainable objectives, and their part in them, the chances of success are much increased. An informal contract in which what the practitioner is able to offer and what the family is willing to do are spelt out is one way of summarising the session. Acknowledgements and thanks come last.

This structure can help practitioner and family alike to deal with issues clearly and productively.

Practitioner communication skills

Communication skills have been dealt with at length in other parts of the book, particularly in Chapter 6. Basic skills of listening, attending, reflecting and empathising are essential. The practitioner can both model effective communication and encourage family members in this. Manor (1984) suggests some simple communication rules which will help promote effective and fruitful discussion. Some of these are summarised below:

Speaking directly
This is modelled at the outset of the type of interview described above when the practitioner addresses each person present regardless of age or capability.

Speaking for themselves
It is important to ensure that each person is not only addressed directly, but has the chance to respond. This can be more difficult

than it sounds if someone else answers first. It requires assertiveness on the part of the practitioner to acknowledge the response, but check it out with the person who was asked in the first place.

Practitioner	'How is your walking now, Mrs W.?
Mr W.	'She's really shaky, needs to use the wheelchair.'
Practitioner	'So your husband is feeling that you really need to be in the wheelchair all the time now. What do you feel about that?'
Mrs W.	'Oh, I don't know, I'd like to keep going a bit longer.'

Once both parties' views are recognised negotiation can take place.

Making 'I' statements

The practitioner can help each person to 'own' their feelings. Often concerns are expressed as criticisms of another person.

Mrs S.	'When he comes back from the Day Centre, he takes out his bad temper on me.'
Practitioner	'How do you feel when that happens?'
Mrs S.	'Upset, and guilty that he's had to go.'

It is easier to work with that unhappiness than with the 'blaming' stance originally taken.

Positive re-phrasing

People often phrase requests for change in other people negatively, expressing the wish that they would stop behaving in a certain way rather than making a positive suggestion about how they might act differently. The practitioner may be able to help to turn such wishes into specific and achievable change.

Mrs P.	'I wish he'd stop interfering now he's home all day.'
Practitioner	'You'd like Mr P. to leave you alone to get on with your chores?'
Mrs P.	'Yes. He means well but. . . .'
Practitioner	'What would you like him to do?'
Mrs P.	'Well I'd be happier if he did the garden like he used to.'

Again, this could form the basis of discussion, whereas an argument about whether or not Mr P. does interfere is unlikely to be very productive.

These basic techniques, and others, can help practitioners to help families to negotiate more freely in difficult situations. One final technique which seems to be worth mentioning is what Watzlawick *et al.* (1974) call 'the gentle art of positive re-framing'. To re-frame a situation or piece of behaviour is to offer an alternative view of it which fits the facts as well as the one held. A practitioner may be able to help a family reinterpret behaviour which they see as problematic and in the process either reduce the significance of that behaviour or help the family to find a different way of handling it.

Mr G.	'Ever since the accident she has become more and more difficult to control. We just don't know what to do with her these days. She's cheeky, untidy, won't wash . . . She was such a good child before this happened.'
Practitioner	'How old is Tracey now?'
Mr G.	'She was 13 last week.'
Practitioner	'Well we know that head injuries can produce behaviour problems, but the other possibility, and may be a more likely one, is that Tracey is growing up and starting to assert herself. Teenagers can be a real headache but adolescence doesn't last for ever!'

This very obvious example gives the family an alternative view of Tracey's behaviour, and one which offers them some hope of managing it. Their current stance is that it cannot be changed. But, you may say, perhaps it is the head injury that is causing the problem. Perhaps it is, but no one can know that with complete certainty and if this alternative perspective defuses the situation, the behaviour may improve anyway!

The other feature of positive re-framing is the effect on the practitioner. Helpers, no less than families, can become stuck and see situations in a way which makes the idea of change unimaginable and which may produce strong negative feeling about continuing work. It is not always essential to share a positive re-frame with a family; it may just be used to help the practitioner adopt a more positive attitude. Relatives who fail to visit a client in some form of residential care are often seen as unloving and neglectful. It is equally possible that they are loving and feel guilty and upset about the situation. One way of minimising this upset is to avoid seeing the person. If helpers take the latter view they will be more likely to feel able to support the family in visiting rather than feeling critical of them for not.

Exercise

- Positive re-framing needs practice. . . .

- Think of as many situations as you can either in work or personal life which could do with re-framing and try and find alternative more positive explanations which fit the facts.
- It may be more fun to do this with a group of people.
- The most important thing to bear in mind is that objective truth is an elusive concept!

Conclusion

Whatever the initial reason for involvement with a family, an awareness of family processes can only improve effectiveness. A family-focused approach requires that helpers have some understanding of the interactional nature of behaviour, that they are aware of the influence of their own experiences, that they can observe carefully, think creatively and communicate clearly. All these issues have been considered in the preceding pages which provide a starting point for helpers who wish to work with families in a more systematic way. Some may also be stimulated to read and explore further the concepts and techniques introduced here. If either of these is the case, the chapter has fulfilled its purpose.

References

Bem, D. (1970) *Beliefs, Attitudes and Human Affairs*. New York: Brooks-Cole.

Bennun, I. (1988) Systems theory and family therapy. In Street, E. and Dryden, W., eds. *Family Therapy in Britain*. pp. 3–22. Milton Keynes: Open University Press.

Burnham, J. (1990) *Family Therapy*. London: Routledge.

Carter, E. and McGoldrick, M. (eds) (1980) *The Family Life Cycle*. New York: Gardner Press.

Haley, J. (1974) *Problem-solving Therapy*. London: Jossey Bass.

Hughes, S., Berger, M. and Wright, L. (1978) The family life cycle and clinical intervention. *Journal of Marriage and Family Counselling*. **5,** 33–40.

Manor, O. (ed) (1984) *Family Work in Action*. London: Tavistock.

Minuchin, S. (1974) *Families and Family Therapy*. London: Tavistock.

Murgatroyd, S. and Woolfe, R. (1985) *Helping Families in Distress*. London: Harper and Row.

Satir, V. (1972) *Peoplemaking*. Palo Alto: Science and Behavior Books.

Thorman, G. (1982) *Helping Troubled Families*. London: Aldine Press.

Watzlawick, P., Weakland, J. and Fisch, R. (1974) *Change: Principles of Problem Formation and Problem Resolution*. New York: Norton.

Chapter 9

Working with groups

Ron Chalk

Introduction

In earlier chapters the discussion of the concept of community care has referred to partnership as being a central plank in the provision of a service. This chapter is about looking at what is required of the practitioner involved in facilitating the development of cooperative and collaborative arrangements amongst those concerned both generally at the agency level, as well as particularly at the level of the recipients.

The setting for these partnership arrangements is the human group which in one form or another provides the forum for the meeting of professionals, volunteers, carers and service users. It is in the group that each can outline what they bring to the forum, what their needs are, and what expectations they have of others within the partnerships. Whether the forum takes the shape of a committee, a case conference, an informal meeting of interested parties, or any variation in between, its format and operation will follow the same basic principles and have the same features that make any group what it is, a unique blend of all the characteristics of its members multiplied by the effects of their interaction, which gives rise to the notion that any group is more than the sum total of the individuals that comprise it. It is the professional worker who has an understanding of these principles and is able to tune in to the processes involved who will be able to operate to best effect.

The range of knowledge and skills which are required for effective intervention by the professional practitioner in group situations, commonly referred to as groupwork, is what will be explored together with some guidelines on the way in which it is possible, with a little practice, to acquire the skills and use the knowledge to become more effective in working with groups.

A theoretical foundation

Groupwork takes as its starting point the fact that man is a gregarious, a group animal; that each individual has a need for the company of other individuals and that a coming together of individuals to form a human group is the almost inevitable consequence of human encounter. This basic characteristic is fundamental to the generally accepted notion of the socialisation process in which human beings become what they are in social and emotional terms, as a result of the various group experiences which each has. It commences in the family group, and covers all the formal and informal coming togethers with others in play, school, recreation, work and other endeavours in which people encounter one another.

Each of these experiences contributes something to the formation and development of the individual in terms of knowledge about self and others and helps in understanding and evaluating the part that such relationship play in life, for as Wilson and Ryland said way back in 1949:

> Human beings can be understood only in relation to other human beings. What a man is, is reflected by the behaviour of other men towards him. What a man thinks of himself is his judgement of the reactions of other men to him. The behaviour of any individual is a mirror of his total life-experience, most of which is in groups.

It is in these various group situations too, that some understanding of the social order is developed. It involves awareness of the patterns of organisation which determine the way things are done and about the importance of acknowledging the role and status of members, the norms of behaviour, the beliefs and values which prevail in each group (collectively referred to as group culture). As well as meeting the need for a degree of conformity as a condition of membership, all contribute to a knowledge of the social world.

Along with this developing understanding of human social activity, these experiences provide an opportunity for the individual to practice and develop skills in making and managing relationships, and in seeing them as fulfilling particular needs and functions, according to the circumstances and the people involved. In addition, a shared interest, issue or concern gives a focus for collective group activity, as well as giving a purpose to their involvement with other like-minded individuals.

If one is looking for evidence of the potential effectiveness of groupwork as a method of intervention it may be found in the assumption that if we have become what we are as a result of our previous group experiences, then it would seem feasible that further group experiences consciously set up and managed may change the current state (Douglas 1975).

Groupwork explored

The wide range of group experiences that individuals have helps prepare them to function more or less effectively in the variety of group situations that may be encountered, and to that extent everyone may regard themselves as a potential groupworker. But to be able to use groupwork as a part of a portfolio of professional techniques requires further appraisal and development which may involve un-learning some of what has been acquired within earlier socialisation.

A key factor in the effectiveness of group activity rests in the extent to which those involved feel a commitment towards others in the partnerships as well as to the task which collectively is to be tackled. For the professional practitioner it also requires a confidence in the processes at work, and recognition that these will be most productive if he or she is able to minimise the centrality of the role, especially in terms of its impact on the task activity. In doing this, however, the practitioner may experience frustration and a lack of self fulfilment, unless there is identified some other basis for activity and assessment, since it contrasts so markedly with normal member participation in a group.

As ordinary participants in a group we are socialised into expecting that we have to make known our personal needs, then negotiate alongside others for a recognition and meeting of these needs, and that fulfilment will come from the extent to which they are recognised and met. In contrast, the professional may have to put to one side some personal needs, especially where having them met may deprive other members in the group.

To give an example, we have all experienced the warm glow of satisfaction which comes from being able to say or do something which is valued and admired by others in a group, and in doing so benefit from the gain in status and self worth in relation to that group. It would be easy for the practitioner, given professional knowledge and expertise, together with ascribed status, to maintain and secure a monopoly on that kind of experience and thus to reinforce the perceived superiority which comes from being a professional amongst non-professionals.

If the practitioner is concerned to maximise the use of group resources, it is important that group members are helped to increase self worth and confidence in their own ideas and abilities. This being so, it requires a more conscious use of the self by the practitioner, who assesses the situation on the basis outlined earlier; decides on the response which is most likely to encourage and facilitate members involvement in group activity, and in their contributing towards the group's identified aims. This response may be likened to the role of a catalyst, an agent of change or development.

In helping to actively redress the power balance in the group, the practitioner communicates a recognition that knowledge and expertise take various forms and are not the sole province of the professional, who, as an individual, contributes only one perspective on any problem. For, who can know better about the difficulties of coping with the after-effects of a stroke than the stroke victim and the carers involved; who can know better about the difficulties associated with independent living for the disabled person, than the person experiencing it and the people offering support?

In these as in many other situations, the experience and perceptions of those involved, whether as carers, clients or volunteers, represent a valuable resource for others, undertaking such a task. It helps to equip them, often in a more relevant context, with knowledge, skills and confidence as well as providing a perception of the problems which they could never get from the professional. It helps increase the self worth and status of those contributing which can be an important therapeutic experience in itself.

In all of this, the practitioner's fulfilment, rather than coming from involvement in direct service giving activity, is replaced by the satisfaction of watching those involved become more able, more confident and better equipped to contribute to meeting their own needs.

Acquiring the ability to use this kind of approach with groups is not easy for many people because training may well have emphasised dominance by the professionals in the working partnerships, as well as encouraging a very task-centred focus to professional activity. In contrast, this approach in many cases will be more time consuming, because of the need to move at the pace dictated by group members, as well as sometimes being frustrating because members may want to do things in ways which appear inefficient or inappropriate to the practitioner. But experience suggests that it is the approach which is most likely to get non-professionals involved in the decision-making and provision-making activity which is central to greater independence and to self help.

The skills involved

A reorientation of practitioner activity can begin by developing a commitment to speaking less and looking more. Speaking less gives space for more thinking and encourages more listening; looking more encourages the development of purposeful observation. Both these basic activities will increase the perceptive skills and abilities of the practitioner, which may only have developed to the level required for everyday social involvement, where casual awareness of group interaction almost at the subconscious level is sufficient.

For the professional worker these skills are a key element in the helping process where the continual making and updating of assessments about the needs and resources of group members is necessary. This requires a conscious effort to perceive and interpret activity against a background of what is known both about the group generally, and the individuals that make it up, in terms of their strengths, needs, motivations and characteristics. It is the interaction of all these factors which create the processes and give the group its dynamic properties.

Groupwork might be described as consisting of the conscious and deliberate observation and utilisation of the group process, for purposes of maximising group resources. If this is to be undertaken effectively, it requires practice by the practitioner, in everyday situations, to increase ability to undertake it purposefully but inconspicuously, so as to maintain a natural involvement in group-life; in effect, to practice being a participant observer.

Exercise

Try this out after contact with a group. Start by noting down as much about what went on as possible: who was present, how they each behaved, and what effect it had on other individuals, and the group generally. Then find someone else who was also involved and share the notes, comments etc. with them, to see if they perceived it in the same way.

There may be differences in what was seen and remembered, reflecting the level of observation skill of you and others involved. It is also likely that there will be differences in the interpretation of events. This is because interpretation is bound up with the personal construct of events.

These differences should be explored and discussed to see what can be learnt. It should be noted that since it is largely personal interpretation which determines behaviour, the individual's current understanding of events will remain a valid basis for action; to try to respond on the basis of another person's interpretation would inevitably lead to problems.

The exercise should emphasise that the aim for the group practitioner is not only to increase observational skills but also to improve knowledge and understanding of groups and individuals. This will provide a broader base upon which to make an interpretation of events. Together these will increase awareness and enable a more conscious and measured response by the practitioner to the variety of group situations encountered. In turn, this increased awareness can be used to help members undertake activities which lead to the meeting of individual and group needs.

Some features of groups

Different groups will have features in common, but they will also differ in some aspects of their make up and operation, and recognising these similarities and differences is important for the practitioner.

The first thing to note is that a collection of individuals can only be regarded as a group when they have some common purpose, some activity, interest or concern, that they wish to jointly pursue. It is only when they express their expectations of the group experience and, through this, identify the similarities or at least a compatibility in their needs, that they begin to develop some group identity. It is the identifying of this shared purpose which gives the group a focus for the many tasks which it has to undertake in order to achieve its objectives. To facilitate a task, there is the other much less explicit, but equally important, activity of providing the means for cooperation and sharing; namely, the communication and interaction between members, often referred to as the process dimension.

These two dimensions, *task* and *process*, both require attention by the group and the practitioner, though, by their very nature, the social processes are more difficult for the group. This is where the practitioner, as a facilitator, will have an important part to play in the context of the role described earlier. Problems such as communication blockage or breakdown, as well as more general issues about interaction, will need to be explored not just in terms of effect, but also of underlying causes.

The task and process dimensions apply to all groups, but in addition there are features which can attach to different kinds of group and practitioner awareness. Understanding of these will help towards a more harmonious working with the group. Amongst these are such things as origins of the group, degree of structure and formality, and nature of membership.

Origins of the group

This refers to whether the group is natural or was formed for a particular purpose. An example of a natural group is a peer group consisting of people who have come together, perhaps spontaneously, because they have something in common which leads them to feel exclusive and self-contained, e.g. age, background, country of origin, which may give them a reason for their collective being. Unless the practitioner shares the characteristics it may well be difficult to establish a working base. A formed group, on the other hand, may be thought of as having been consciously planned and set up to meet some explicit and identified need, e.g. to organise a particular event or to offer help and support to a particular group of people. If the practitioner is not involved from the outset, then acceptance may be gained if: an acknowledgement of the need is expressed; some indication of practitioner contribution can be given; and the group is recognised as worthwhile by its members.

Degree of structure and formality

If the practitioner is involved from the outset, it may be possible to influence development, but if not, then account needs to be taken of the ground rules for operation of the group. These rules may vary from a formal constitution (a kind of bureaucratised culture) to a set of simple guidelines, which may specify things like duties attached to set roles; a particular way of taking and implementing decisions, and offering guidelines or rules governing the acquisition and use of resources. These factors will certainly affect, and perhaps limit, the extent to which the practitioner is able to encourage personal development and initiative amongst members. Common examples of such groups may be the local branch of a national voluntary organisation (e.g. Spastics Society) or a specialist sub-group of a more broadly based local welfare group (e.g. Council of Community Service).

Open or closed membership

This final aspect of group life is one which has implications for the culture of the group. One important way which all groups, formal and informal, have of passing on their culture is through communication between members. If membership is transient, as in an 'open' group, then communication may well be limited and therefore group culture may not be very stable. This can lead to lack of clarity about ends (purpose) and means (agreed ways of doing things) in the group. Here the practitioner may need to act as a link in the communication chain at times when uncertainty occurs. However, care needs to be taken to ensure that this is not used as a back-door way of imposing change which has not been agreed by members, though it may be a chance to get members to review and, if desired, openly change any aspects of the group's culture.

Identifying needs in the group

The basis of any service is identifying the needs of likely recipients and setting up a programme to meet those needs. In groupwork, whilst the needs of the individual remain paramount, there are needs related to the task and process areas of the group which also have to be considered. The success of the programme for individuals is very much bound up with the effectiveness of task and process activity. To emphasise their interdependence they are often depicted as three interlocking circles (see Figure 9.1).

Before considering the particular needs of an individual member of the group, it is important to recognise that all individuals have a generalised range of needs in common and one way of thinking about these is in terms of Maslow's hierarchy (Maslow 1962). This suggests that human needs can be seen as having an ascending order of priority which starts with the very basic physical needs and ascends up to the need for self-actualisation (see Figure 9.2).

Maslow further suggests that lower order needs have to be met before middle and higher order needs can be properly fulfilled. Since a principal component of groupwork is social interaction – a middle order need in the hierarchy – it is important to recognise that people will not get the best out of a group situation if they are cold, hungry or tired, or feeling insecure or unsafe, for whatever reason. Any organisational arrangement will have to ensure that these basic needs are met by group activity, or by whatever other means seems appropriate, before an attempt is made to meet any other particular and personal needs which may have been identified.

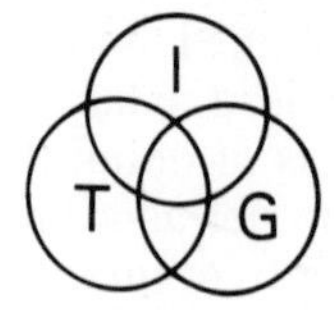

Where I = individual

T = task

G = process (or group maintenance)

Figure 9.1 Group interdependence

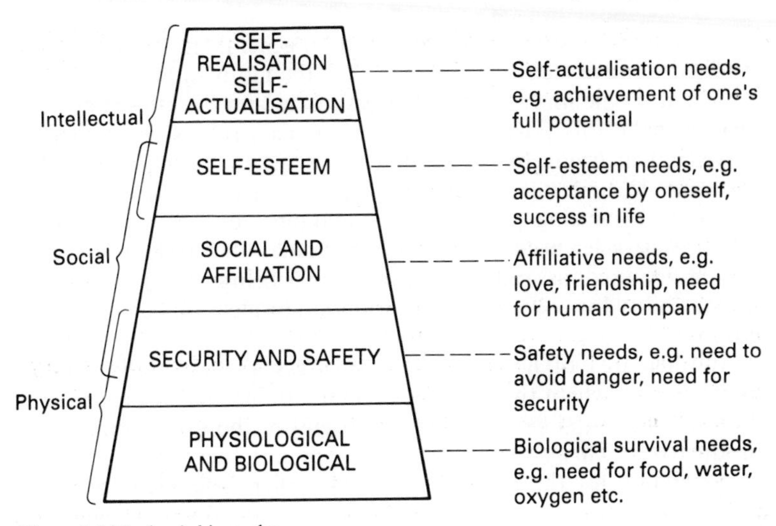

Figure 9.2 Maslow's hierarchy

Individuals needs

The assessment of individual needs are undertaken in accordance with normal professional procedures related to the physical, psychological and social self. The outcomes are used to formulate objectives and a plan of action. The decision to use groupwork as the forum for intervention has, however, to be based on whether it is possible and practical to meet these needs in a group setting, or whether a more traditional one-to-one approach might be more appropriate. This decision relies on: the professional assessment of the nature of the need; what is known about the particular individuals concerned, in terms of their social and psychological demeanour at the time; and whether the individuals are likely to be able to acknowledge and share the commonality of need required, to produce a viable cohesive unit. If people cannot identify with the objectives and goal of the group, they are unlikely to want to work together to plan and implement action proposals.

Task needs

Tasks are the needs concerned directly with the goal of the group, and include such things as ensuring that everyone has a common understanding of what is intended and, in general terms, of what is required to advance the goal, as well as the motivation to want to achieve it. Some knowledge of the resources and facilities is necessary to make this possible. The practitioner's role is again facilitative, but in trying to ensure that these tasks are met, it may be necessary to undertake some direct goal-centred activity such as providing a meeting place, and tea-making facilities (which may meet lower order needs also). Perhaps some other basic resources may be required, as well as the practitioner being prepared to take responsibility for collection of information or ideas on behalf of the group.

Another area of need is that of process and especially group maintenance, where the focus is on maintaining the efficient operation of the social processes so as to ensure the group functions productively. This is the area where the practitioner will have most responsibility for the reasons indicated earlier. This includes such things as ensuring, as far as possible, a stress-free environment where people can feel at ease with one another, and where they enter into interaction freely and willingly. Also, given that communication is a central part of process activity, it includes checking to ensure that intended meanings are shared by all, which requires the clarifying of technical language and jargon where it occurs. In addition, it involves getting the group to investigate any 'hidden agendas' which may emerge. These can be very distracting, possibly even destructive of group activity if ignored. Their existence quite often indicates an undisclosed personal need which, wherever possible, should be incorporated into the overall goal of the group, and thus become part of the 'official' agenda.

Exercise

Think about a group that you have had recent contact with, and list the needs under the headings 'individual', 'task' and 'process'. Are there needs which you have listed which do not appear to have been met? What is the effect on the individuals and or group, of this deprivation?

Stages in the life of the group

A group can be thought of as going through various stages in its life. These have been described by Tuckman (1965) as *forming, storming, norming* and *performing*, and at each stage particular needs may be more in evidence.

At the forming stage, when people are just getting together, individual needs prevail. People may be uncertain about themselves, and their place in the group. They are likely to feel insecure and want to be assured that they will fit in, and their needs will be met.

At the storming stage, there is much discussion and negotiation about what the group is to be set up for, what boundaries and constraints it may be subject to, who the leaders will be, and how they will serve the group. At this stage, there is still some emphasis on personal needs, but also increasingly on process needs.

At the norming stage, individual needs begin to give way to task as well as process needs, as the group get down to the business of sorting out the rules (norms) for operation, who is going to do what, and how it will be done. This will involve more discussion about roles, including leadership, and about relationships within the group.

The performing stage is marked by a degree of stability with emphasis on task activity, and members working well as a cooperative unit.

Using the model of the three interlocking circles, the emphasis at the various stages can be depicted by the size of circle, shown in Figure 9.3.

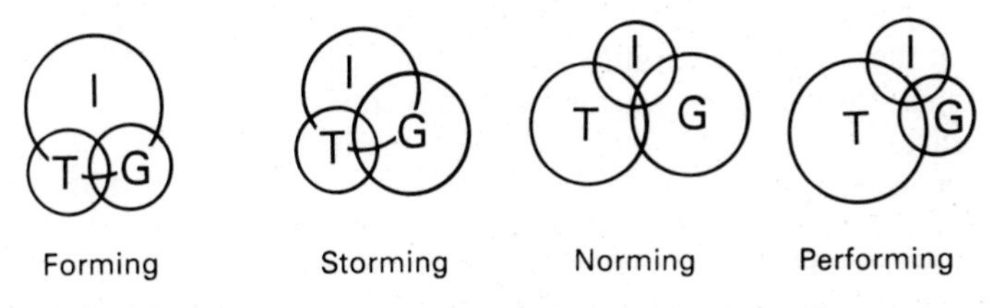

Figure 9.3 Group interlocking (where I = individual, T = task and G = process or group maintenance)

It is important to remember that these stages are not self contained, and also that any group is likely to move back as well as forward during its lifetime. For instance, such things as the introduction of a new member, or the identifying of a fresh objective, as well as challenges to the norms, or competition for leadership, are all likely to result in the group reverting to the storming and norming phase, before stabilising and moving back to performing again.

Exercise

Think again about a group you have had recent contact with, and construct the three circle diagram to indicate at what stage of development you think they have reached.

Meeting needs in the group

So far, the discussion has been about what kinds of need may exist in a group, and what practitioner activity is required to identify and, where appropriate, meet these needs. However, since a central tenet of groupwork is to maximise the use of group resources, and through this increase self help and independence. A way is needed to think about how individuals in groups can make a greater contribution. The concept of role can provide this.

A role can be thought of as an expected pattern of behaviour of someone holding a particular position in a group or organisation. It can be formalised by being given a title, e.g. Manager. This brings with it an ascribed status, which is assigned by the body appointing the person to the role. This will involve the role holder in a power relationship with any other person in the group or organisation based on their relative positions in the heirarchy and creates opportunities for the exercise of influence. The potential for a power relationship may also exist where someone is appointed to a professional position, which involves working with lay people, or volunteers, and who is seen by them as having an authority. This is by virtue of their perceived ability to carry out functional activity which will benefit the group, as was briefly commented on previously.

In earlier discussion, reference was made to the idea of the member as a group resource. In role terms, it can be seen that any member may earn a status, bringing with it a chance to influence others, if the group regards their contribution as beneficial. The practitioner can do much to help the group evaluate activity, by assigning roles with their attendant responsibilities, which will contribute to the meeting of identified needs. The practitioner does this by ensuring consensus on objectives, agreeing the functional activity required to meet them, and then, on the basis of previous knowledge and current observation, create opportunities for group-based resources to be made available in response to need. To give an example, if the practitioner knows that someone in the group has experience in the home care of a stroke patient, then when an aspect of that experience would seem to be of use to the group, the practitioner attempts to facilitate its sharing by the member with the group. In doing this, the practitioner enhances the members' status and thus their influence. This leads to greater self fulfilment, and this in turn increases their commitment to the group.

Exercise

Think of a recent occasion when you observed someone facilitating member activity in a group in this way. Can you also think of occasions when you could have enabled this to happen, but did not? What would you do differently to help someone share their experience, for the benefit of the group?

The practitioner's role

Earlier references were made to the nature of the practitioner's role, and how the relationships with members of the group may best be understood and used. This section is about the activities and techniques involved. It is important, though, to acknowledge that group practitioner activity may be complicated by being combined with other roles, mostly commonly that of agency representative and to consider how the practitioner can handle this.

Take the example of a practitioner employed by a health authority which is also a partner in a project: the authority will expect that any resources they make available will be accompanied by representation on any decision-making body set up to administer it. If the practitioner is there in that role also, this should be discussed with the group at an early stage to clarify the situation and to make known the resource commitments of the agency. This will ensure that the practitioner's position is not compromised by suggestions of hidden bias. When discussion about resources subsequently occurs, the practitioner should then be able to contribute more clearly in the role of representative.

Potential complication is that of leadership. The role of group practitioner could easily be regarded as synonymous with that of the group leader. Some may say that it is inevitably so, particularly in a situation where it is a professional working with lay people and volunteers. However, it is important for the democratic operation of the group that the practitioner does not allow this situation to develop, but rather encourages the view that leadership may move around the group according to the activity of individual members.

Since leadership is about leaders influencing followers, it is possible to regard a range of functional activity as leader activity, to the extent that it influences other members and thus the course of events in the group. As such it may be regarded as functional leadership. And so the person 'holding the stage' at any one point may be regarded as the leader of the moment, rather than leadership always being seen to rest with the practitioner, with all the power that this implies.

Bales (1950) has identified some of the more common individual activities which may be associated with functional leadership. They are categorised according to the area of group activity that they serve. He defines task activity as consisting of the following functions:

Initiating activity
Proposing solutions, suggesting new ideas, new definitions of the problem, new attack on the problem or new organisation of material.

Seeking information
Asking for clarification of suggestions, requesting additional information or facts.

Seeking opinions
Looking for an expression of feeling about something from member seeking clarification of values, suggestions or ideas.

Giving information
Offering facts or generalisations, relating one's own experience to the group's problem to illustrate points.

Giving opinions
Stating an opinion or belief concerning a suggestion(s), particularly concerning its value rather than its factual basis.

Elaborating
Clarifying, giving examples or developing meanings, trying to envisage how a proposal might work if adopted.

Coordinating
Showing relationships among various ideas or suggestions, putting ideas or suggestions together.

Summarising
Restating suggestions or ideas after discussion, stating the group's position at a given point.

Group maintenance activity, which Bales defines as consisting of functions required in strengthening and maintaining group processes and activities, includes:

Encouraging
Being friendly, warm, responsive to others, praising others and their ideas, agreeing with and accepting the contributions of others.

Gate-keeping
Helping all to contribute, keeping the group to its task.

Standard setting
Expressing group standards for use in choosing its content, procedures or decisions.

Expressing group feeling
Summarising what group feeling is sensed to be, describing reactions of group to ideas.

A third category is that which spans both task and process, and includes:

Evaluating
Measuring accomplishments against goals and standards of group.

Diagnosing
Determining sources of difficulties and appropriate next steps. Analysing blocks to progess.

Testing for consensus
Asking for group opinion to see if decision is near, sending up trial balloons.

Mediating
Harmonising, conciliating differences, making compromises.

Relieving tension
Draining off tension through joking or changing context.

All of these activities should be regarded by the practitioner as potential opportunities for member involvement, and to be seen to be fulfilling leadership needs in a real and productive way, as well as shifting the focus from the practitioner.

Exercise

The next time you are in a group, try identifying the activities of members in terms of the categories and functions listed by Bales above. Can you perceive the activities in leadership terms, i.e. that the person performing the activity is the 'leader of the moment', and as such is influencing others and thus the course of events in the group?

The concern with group leadership, reinforced by the earlier discussion about skills, indicates practitioner activity falling into three broad areas. First and foremost, there is the monitoring activity, which involves observing and making assessments about individuals and the group in terms of its needs and responses. Second, there is the enabling and facilitating activity, which may be thought of as 'oiling the cogs' of group life to make it possible for members to be involved according to their needs and interests, especially in relation to communication relationships and resource issues. Third, there is direct service-giving activity, related to the identified task of the group, and it is this area which is perhaps the most challenging for the practitioner. If the response is too 'generous' in terms of what is done, it may undermine attempts to encourage the group's independence and yet, if it is too limited, it may create a level of frustration which could be damaging to the group, as well as affecting the practitioner's credibility. A measured response is required, involving a conscious use of self based on the practitioner's assessment of the group capacity to meet its own needs.

Batten (1967) describes a model of working which he calls the directive/non-directive approach. In this the practitioner constantly monitors the state of the group in terms of its resources and its self-help abilities and responds in a flexible way according to the assessment of need along a scale from the 'directive', which involves the practitioner in making all the decisions, and undertaking all the functions required for the group, to the 'non-directive', in which the practitioner makes no contribution to group activity, and is involved only in monitoring the group's performance.

Clearly, in practice, the situation is likely to be ever-changing, both within one group meeting as well as from meeting to meeting. This emphasises the need for the practitioner to be flexible in response to these changing needs, and to see directive–non-directive as two ends of a continuum, within which practitioner activity takes place. This is illustrated in Figure 9.4.

Batten emphasises that this approach can only be used effectively by the practitioner who is firmly committed to a democratic model

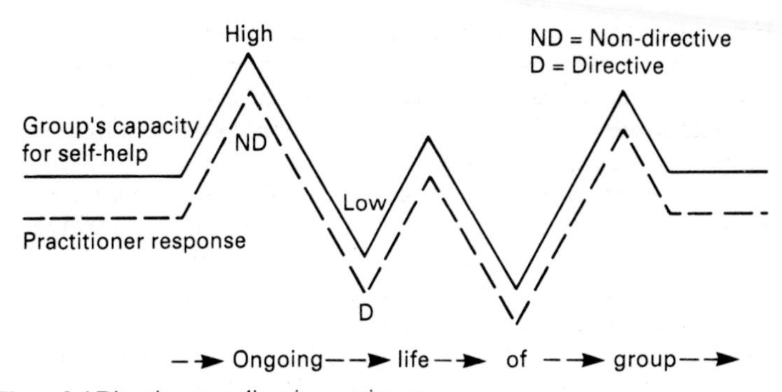

Figure 9.4 Directive–non-directive continuum

of working, in which the group has rights as well as responsibilities in relation to identifying and meeting its own needs. This emphasises the importance of observation and interpretation as being central to the effective use of the techniques.

Exercise

What is your customary way of operating in a group? Are you able to be flexible and measured in your responses to member activity? Try to monitor your approach, and to be more conscious of the effects of your responses in terms of the apparent willingness and ability of members to contribute to meeting needs. Ask a colleague how they perceive the impact which you, the professional practitioner, have on a group.

Diagnosing and dealing with group problems

Within the life of any group, situations will arise which challenge its smooth running. It is important to see these as an intrinsic part of group life. The whole process of development from forming to performing consists of a series of challenges which the group has to deal with and which cannot be avoided if the group is going to mature and become task functional. There are occasions when the nature of a challenge, especially from individuals involved in what Bales (1950) calls 'non-functional activity' carried out for self-centred reasons, is not only non-productive but perhaps even destructive. It thus becomes a problem. It is when this kind of situation arises that the practitioner may have to consider a greater degree of direct intervention, depending on the assessment of the group ability to deal with it.

The range of challenging activity which might be considered productive is anything which stimulates constructive action, or assists with creating cohesion or encourages commitment to the group and its ideals. The questioning of group aims, or of the way the group is using its resources may come into this category. On the other hand, such things as scapegoating of an individual, or the deliberate undermining of group activity by an uncooperative

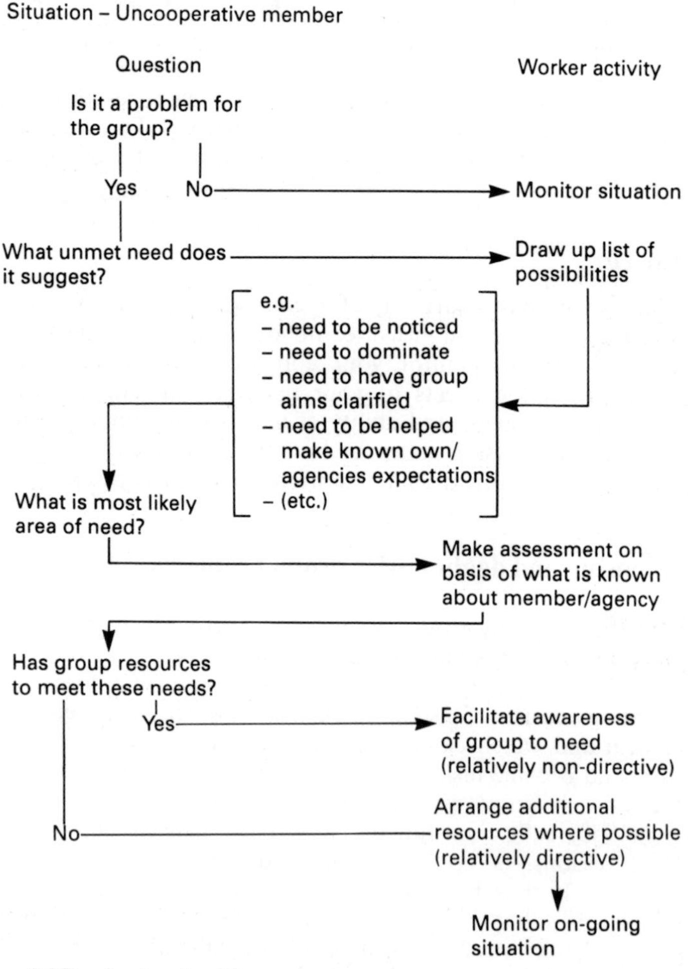

Figure 9.5 Step-by-step algorithm

member, may be considered non-productive in group terms, and perhaps destructive of the individuals involved. These require more directive practitioner action. It is important to remember, however, that all the circumstances need to be fully considered in interpreting a particular event or situation. What may in one circumstance be regarded as scapegoating, may in other circumstances be interpreted as a quite legitimate use of group pressure by the group. Similarly, the withholding of a particular known resource by an individual or sub-group may be seen as obstructive, but may on the other hand be regarded as just the stimulus the group needs to get it to examine the commitment of its members.

The key to making an accurate assessment of the situation again depends upon the practitioner's knowledge of the group and the individuals within it. One approach is to consider the presenting behaviour in the context of needs being expressed, and needs being met, as described earlier. Anything identified as problematic may be seen as an expression of unmet needs. The role of the practitioner consists of identifying the needs and providing as much assistance as seems necessary to enable those needs to be met in the most constructive way possible.

It may help to understand this approach by taking as an example the uncooperative member, and presenting it step-by-step as a simple algorithm (Figure 9.5).

It is possible to assess needs, and formulate a practitioner response to many of the difficulties that may be encountered in a group, not just in relation to the individual but also to task and process need. Some difficulties may require a more extended analysis, depending on the presenting situation. This approach should help the practitioner to avoid feeling helpless in what might otherwise be experienced as an overwhelming situation.

Exercise

Identify the last challenging group situation that you faced, and work through the algorithm. Are there any aspects of your situation that are not covered? What other questions might the practitioner need to ask in order to take account of these?

Principles into practice

It may be useful to conclude by looking briefly at the steps involved in a piece of practical groupwork. It should be regarded as a recipe of ingredients, rather than a blueprint for action.

The process usually starts with someone becoming aware of unmet needs, either of their own, or of others for whom they may have a concern or interest. This awareness is shared with other people, and as a result they get together, and talk about what they can do to try to meet the needs. It is at this point that the presence of a professional practitioner with some responsibility for the areas of the need concerned may help those involved to organise themselves, by discussing with them what is the best way forward.

The first requirement will be to clarify the needs and to ensure a measure of consensus about what should be done, and whether an action group is the best way of achieving it. If agreement is reached, then the next step is to formulate aims and objectives which provide a framework for action. These should be expressed in a way which is understandable to everyone and preferably in action terms which will enable them to be used to assess progress in the desired areas.

This should be followed by an action plan which covers:

- the roles and responsibilities of those involved;
- the resources available, what will have to be acquired, and from where;
- the time scale, with targets for various stages in the plan and any priorities identified;
- any constraints, which may interface with the planned activity, together with some indication of how they may be dealt with.

These items provide the basis for both an initial meeting, and an ongoing agenda to review developments. Practitioner activity has to be concerned with supporting and monitoring progress, in the process as well as the task areas, and ensuring that individuals are gaining fulfilment from their involvement. The monitoring activity will be assisted by simple written recordings based on observations of the groups activities. This will enable the practitioner to build up a picture of developments in the various areas and indicate where any additional resources or direct input may be required. The recordings will also provide a firmer basis for assessment of progress and evaluation of the project in relation to the aims and objectives set by the group at the outset.

A final exercise

Apply the above guidelines to an actual or potential group-work situation, and then talk it through with a colleague. Pay particular attention to the way you have formulated your aims and objectives (do they reflect the needs as identified?); what about the timescale; is it realistic? (remember, you may be working with people who have little or no previous experience of structured task activity); have you considered *all* the possible constraints (time, money, space, people, attitudes)? Are you clear about how you will help the group evaluate its efforts?

If you have tried the exercise and followed the principles outlined in this chapter, implementing it in practice should lead to a productive and fulfilling experience for all those involved – the providers, the recipients and the practitioner. This is clearly an important requirement in any collaborative venture and a key to the successful use of groupwork in community care.

References

Bales, R. F. (1950) *Interaction Process Analysis*. Cambridge, Mass: Addison Wesley.
Douglas, T. (1981) *Groupwork Practice*. London: Tavistock.
Maslow, A. H. (1962) *Towards a Psychology of Being*. New York: Van Nostrand.
Tuckman, B. W. (1965) Developmental sequences in small groups *Psychological Bulletin*, **63**(6), 384–399.
Wilson, G. and Ryland, G. (1949) *Social Group Work Practice*. Boston: Houghton Mifflin.

Further reading

Prestoon-Shoot, M. (1987) *Effective Groupwork*. London: Macmillan Education.

Chapter 10

Working in the community

Ann Compton

Organisational structures

This chapter considers the factors which influence how any service is delivered in the community. The issues addressed are relevant to all community practitioners. Although examples are particularly related to health and physiotherapy it is not intended to address clinical detail, since practitioners will find that this is common practice wherever located. The background knowledge and skills' development which have been mentioned in previous chapters will impinge upon professional practice in the community, together with influences affecting the way a local community organises itself.

Organisational influences

Whatever services are offered in and to a community, whether national or local, they all come under similar influences, although some will have more bearing on one particular service than another. How each service is organised and operates will also have an effect on any other service. The interdependence of health, social, education and voluntary services and some of the influences upon them need consideration, together with the effect of change in any of the services' organisation and operation, or that of any influencing factor as shown in Figure 10.1.

Exercise

The largest local employer closes, causing half the working population to be unemployed. Which other factors in Figure 10.1 will be affected?

Key services in community care

It is not intended to review or describe these services comprehensively since an up-to-date review of all the social services is published

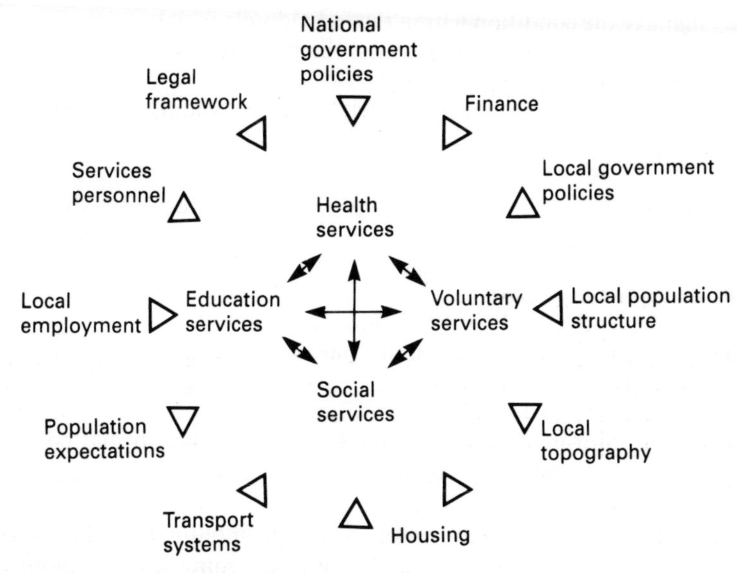

Figure 10.1 Interdependence of services

annually by the Family Services Association. The purpose is to raise matters which impinge upon community practice.

Health services

Ninety per cent of health care takes place outside the hospitals, provided through primary health care and community health services.

Primary health care, focused upon general practice, is the contact point for individuals with 'dis-ease', either from pain, altered function, worry or a visible problem (swelling, rash, cut), and pregnancy or family planning needs. Originally solely a doctor in practice, over the years the primary health care team has evolved, each member playing a part in fulfilling the brief of the general practitioner. This is to cure, manage, educate about and prevent 'dis-ease' in the physical, psychological and social aspects of life so that the quality of that life is improved or eased.

To achieve this the doctor and all the team members need to be able to:

- select the 'real' disease from the minor complaint;

- manage the condition within the individual's social setting;
- know where and how to find further information to assist management;
- know when and why to refer, and to whom, for specific assistance.

Community health services are responsible for local health provision, including:

- its maintenance;
- the prevention of ill health within the locality;
- improving the local community's health;
- promoting health strategies;
- collecting local data affecting health;
- giving information, advice and guidance on health matters to both public and private bodies.

Service such as health education, health promotion, pre-schol and school health, immunisation and family planning are commonly offered, and provisions made to meet 'port of entry' (to the country) health requirements.

Exercise

A child who has just returned from abroad is taken ill at school. This is diagnosed as typhoid fever. Consider the public health implications and the role of the local community health department.

Social services

Local provision is greatly influenced by the statutory obligations which must be met. The Acts of Parliament from which these statutes derive are concerned with child care and safety, mental health and disabled persons. These Acts include discretionary clauses – 'may' – alongside statutory – 'must'. It is the discretionary clauses which allow the variations found in service provisions, and which are dependent upon the many local influencing factors. This is why people are sometimes disappointed in their expectations of the assistance which is available to them. Clauses within new Acts may not all become statutes at the same time, which can cause raised hopes to be dashed.

Exercise

A newly disabled woman living alone in rented accommodation needs the following to be fully independent and have the quality of life that she wishes: grab rails and hi-lo bath seat in the bathroom, domestic help, help-call telephone, discretionary parking, word processing skills for re-employment, downstairs toilet facilities, meals on wheels, access to swimming and social club facilities. Which of these will be provided by her Local Authority? How would her needs be met in your own locality?

Education services

Local Authority provision has to be made for all children of school age, 5 to 16, and for those with special needs from 2 to 21 if it is considered necessary. Once a child is identified as having special needs assessment is made by Health, Social and Education services, resulting in a statement being written which defines those needs and what action is necessary to enable the child to optimise his or her potential. Provision must then be made to ensure that the requirements in the statement are met. Parental choice must also be taken into consideration. Parental expectations will be influenced by both family and neighbourhood values and expectations.

With the move away from special schools towards the integration of all children into their local schools the working together of health, social and education services is often required to achieve a balance between the needs of the statemented child and those of the other children in the school.

Exercise

A wheelchair user lives equidistant from two schools. One school has already been adapted for another child, but his parents wish him to attend the other school, which holds some classes upstairs. The parents consider that it should be possible for the school to be organised so that their son has the education that they choose. Consider the likely solutions, and the implications on financial resources, the staff, the parents, the boy and the other schoolchildren of each of your solutions.

Voluntary services

Community care relies heavily on the use of volunteers, whether as individuals helping at home or as groups of helpers working in clubs or day centres. Some volunteers may be involved in fundraising or in organisation rather than at the 'coal face', but all are people with concern to fill gaps in provisions of the official services. Some voluntary services are nationally organised whilst others are very local. They vary as to the:

- scope of the organisation;
- types of services offered;
- method of delivery;
- targeting of the group to be assisted.

Targeting may be by age, medical condition, social grouping, locality, individual or occupational background.

Examples

A blind person obtains talking books from the Royal National Institute for the Blind, but receives the local news from a small band of volunteers who produce and circulate tapes to members of the local Blind Club.

A woman with multiple sclerosis has received information leaflets from the Multiple Sclerosis Society and belongs to the local MS group for social activities and support. Her one previous acquaintance who has MS does not attend this group as he lives outside its catchment and transport area.

A terminal cancer patient might have night nursing support from the Macmillan Nursing Service, a weekly grant for the additional heating from the National Society for Cancer Relief, meals on wheels delivered by the WRVS and the local churches' Good Neighbour scheme providing help with shopping and visiting.

A disabled young man has a place at university but the size of the campus and its hills are beyond his ability and stamina. Local people join together solely to fundraise for a powered vehicle which he can also transport in his car.

It is the right of an individual to choose whether to use any or all of the state or voluntary provisions or to make their own private arrangements.

Example

A person may choose to use the National Health Service and claim all the social benefits to which they are entitled but prefer to pay for special equipment and home adaptation.

Exercise

- List all the national then local organisations that would be of help to your clients.
- Find out what these organisations can offer.
- Check how to contact or access their services.
- Discover where you can find out about other organisations and their provisions.

If you keep this list to hand and up to date it is a valuable resource when problem solving.

Service parameters

There are many influences which affect the nature of and demand upon all the comunity services. Some of the more important are:

Legal framework

The statutes provide the framework upon which services are based. They lay down the conditions that must be met by the state-provided services as well as indicating the parameters within which the individual services must operate. They designate both the service providers and those who are entitled to benefit from that service.

Exercises

Look at all the Acts of Parliament which have affected community care provision starting with the 1970 The Chronically Sick and Disabled Persons' Act and the 1970 Education Act.

- A 64-year-old is causing considerable concern by his strange daytime behaviour, night-time wandering, self-neglect and threats to his family and friends. What legislation might be invoked?

National government policies

Social policy is essentially determined by political considerations. Politicians will be influenced by:

- Ideological factors, e.g. the belief that a market economy for provision would lead to the encouragement of private initiatives and competitive tendering, but the weakest may be lost from the system. Conversely a command economy, along the lines of Karl Marx, is designed to provide for all but can lead to lack of responsibility and reliance on the 'Nanny State'.

- Financial considerations, e.g. additional social support would require a considerable increase in funding.
- Public opinion, e.g. extra resources may be allocated if public opinion is very strong that children are not being sufficiently protected despite efforts to meet the statutes. The Patients' Charter was introduced because of concern about care within the National Health Service.
- Activity of pressure groups, e.g. support for carers, was included in the National Health Service and Community Care Act 1990 as a result of the activities of organisations such as Age Concern, National Carers' Association and other concerned groups.
- Availability of data, e.g. data about lost working days from accidents at work and their cost to the nation resulted in the Health and Safety at Work Act 1974 and subsequent legislation.

A fuller example of this is the shift in social policy enshrined in the Community Care Act that caring should be freed from its institutional base and many more services be made available in the community.

Historically many caring services have traditionally been provided with the user going to the service instead of the service going to the user. Use has perforce been limited by:

- The accessibility of the service site. Distance, cost and travelling time can be a deterrent for use to both the community practitioner and the service user. There is some evidence that suggests that rural practitioners have tended to refer less to central services than their city counterparts.
- The gatekeeping processes which deter some from seeking help. The need to obtain special forms and their complexity is one process. For physiotherapy within the NHS a general practitioner used to have to refer those needing it to a consultant for physiotherapy to be prescribed. It is only relatively recent that general practitioners have been able to refer patients directly.
- The pattern of delivery such as routines for appointments of transportation, e.g. twice-weekly treatment appointments were only given for Tuesdays and Thursdays although some of the catchment area had no bus service on Thursdays. Hospital transport could only be used for all visits, despite that it only ran twice in the day on a long and circuitous route.
- Appointments only being available in working hours and no

consideration being given to the service users other commitments or responsibilities. Failure to attend may itself become a gatekeeping process as these people may be excluded from claiming rights or be seen as a poor investment.

Example

Every time a consultant saw a child she was referred for physiotherapy but her mother did not take her regularly although all consultant appointments were kept. When visited by a community practitioner, it was found that the mother was also caring for her aunt with senile dementia and her own bed-ridden mother. She was unable to leave the house for more than a few minutes unless someone else was present. The mother was a very retiring person and did not find it easy to get other people to come in three times a week for the 3½ hours an afternoon that it took for her child to attend her 30 minute therapy session. The father took time off work for consultant appointments but lost pay and could not afford to do this for therapy sessions. It was practice that if more than three consecutive appointments were missed without prior notice the appointment time was cancelled and the non-attender placed on the waiting list. When poor attenders were re-referred they were often deemed as having less priority than others. The mother was assidiously carrying out the exercises she had both been taught and seen done by the physiotherapist, as she knew how important they were for her child. Her irregular and non-attendance had given her a reputation as an uncaring mother.

With the changes in the National Health Service of the late 1980s and early 1990s the traditional service providers are having to consider how their treatment policies are affecting rehabilitation services. The intensified use of hospital beds from earlier discharge, day surgery and similar action has helped meet user need, but rehabilitation is often incomplete or post-operative therapy required. Alongside this, more people are being cared for in the community by the primary care team or specialist teams, such as those in mental health, and greater emphasis is being placed on preventive health through health promotion. Physiotherapists are having to look at the distribution of their practice to enable the most effective use of practitioners, the outcome of which might be that staff are focused in the community instead of in the traditional ward and outpatient areas, the shift being determined by local need.

Exercise

Read the Patient's Charter and the Citizen's Charter and consider how they apply to all patients and all citizens and how they might affect your work.

Local service provision

Helping service culture

Services in different areas develop their own culture, which in turn influence the way in which services are delivered. These cultures are derived from the knowledge and attitudes of the personnel who are responsible for service delivery. Even where there are national guidelines there are inevitably wide local variations in the way the service is experienced by consumers. There is constant interaction between the community practitioner and the community in which they work which further modifies the organisational culture.

Service management

The management task is to ensure that a service is delivered efficiently and economically, using both human and material resources effectively.

When developing unit strategy a manager has to consider:

- the previous performance of the service;
- all the organisational influences (see Figure 10.1);
- development opportunities for the service;
- staff potential;
- the identified needs that are to be met.

This analysis enables the manager to set objectives for the service and make realistic plans so that those objectives may be achieved. In large organisations complex management systems will evolve and interpretation of policies will undergo modification as it passes through the system.

Within the National Health Service the Department of Health sets out an overall service plan to meet the health needs of the nation.

Example

In the mid 1980s the Department of Health decided that the best management structure to ensure that its policies would be effectively delivered at local level was to divide the country into regions, which themselves were divided into districts. Guidelines were issued for the management structure at Health District level. These stated that a district general manager should work through a system of unit management. Local interpretation of the guidelines varied. Some general managers decided that the best unit division to meet local need was two or three units, such as community and acute services, based on location. Others opted for units based upon user groups, e.g. paediatrics, mental health, geriatrics, cutting across service locations. Under these systems, apart from the unit managers, there were often individual professional service managers who had contractual arrangements with each unit manager for professional input who also contributed to the policy interpretation.

Under the 1990 National Health Service and Community Care Act, often referred to as NHS reforms, the Health Authority, which includes the old District General Manager, is charged with assessing the needs of the population under its care, and making arrangements to meet those needs. It then establishes contracts with providers to undertake the work, taking into account government guidelines on the provision of services. To make the best use of resources, local health authorities will need to share their plans with the managers of the other social services, considering the effects of intended action on each other, and ensuring that none of those entitled to their services fall outside their provisions.

Example

The government wants to see waiting lists for hip replacements reduced to not more than 3 months within 2 years. Additional funding is being allocated by the Department of Health to achieve this target. Each region will allocate a share of this funding to each Health District.

The District Health Authority will decide from their information sources how many hip operations need to be purchased in that financial year to meet this government guideline. The Health Authority then establishes contracts with providers to undertake this work to the standards which it has set for this procedure.

The service providers have to consider a large number of issues even if the orthopaedic surgeons are available to undertake extra work. Amongst these are:

- operating theatre time, equipment and staffing;
- ward space, staff, equipment, and support services;
- laboratory services;
- blood transfusion services;
- sterile supplies department;
- therapy services;
- outpatient appointments.

Staff training may also be required to ensure those employed have the specialist skills.

The effects are not confined to the hospital. The impact on the community may include extra demand on:

- home nursing services;
- community therapy;
- short term loan of aids for daily living equipment;
- home care services;
- hospital and voluntary transport services.

Each service manager will need to consider the effect upon their service as a whole. Amongst their considerations will be those concerning the effects upon the:

- overall workload;
- individual's workload;
- equipment required;
- service budget;
- quality of service to all patients;
- staff skills.

A service provider is then able to formulate a bid to meet the District Health Authority's requirements.

With the service bids in hand, the District Health Authority plan will be drawn up taking into account other on-going health needs, usually after consultation with Social Services and the Family Health Service Authority, which contracts the general practitioner services. The plan may use District Managed Units, National Health Service Trusts, independent hospitals or other facilities, e.g. from Europe, Social Services or the voluntary sector, or any combination of these. The computations are many, but the result will be based on evaluation of local data which allows the best use of the additional finance allocated, and indicates the constraints upon reaching the objective with the quality of care which underlies all health plans.

Although these factors are not directly under the control of the community practitioner it is important for them to appreciate the knock-on effects of what may appear to be isolated changes in care policy.

Parameters for the practitioner

Factors which influence the practitioner are:

Changes in professional status

In physiotherapy professional autonomy, introduced in the early 1980s, altered the professional relationship with medical practitioners. Referral is no longer prescriptive but interprofessional. The physiotherapist uses clinical diagnostic skills to decide appropriate intervention and case management. It has taken time for both the medical practitioners and the physiotherapists to adjust to the different relationship with its different expectations.

Professional experience

Physiotherapy is a profession which works across medical specialties. All physiotherapists are equipped with basic skills, but specific interests develop in post-qualifying practice. A therapist may choose to specialise in neurology rather than acute injuries or paediatrics.

Personal life experience

Each person's life experience influences their attitudes, interpretation of situations and their interactions with other people.

Expectations of interprofessional cooperation

These may be derived from:

- previous experience from a similar post;
- experience as a user,
- hearsay from other users or professionals.

These expectations influence the contribution made and the value placed upon others' work.

Communication network

Communication between different service practitioners can help to build accurate expectations and break down misconceptions. Poor communication usually results in a poor service to the user. Good communication depends upon the:

Possibility of contact
This depends upon the practitioner being aware of whom to contact and where to make that contact.

Ease of contact
Knowing how to make contact and when a person is likely to be available for face-to-face or telephone discussion avoids unnecessary delay and frustration for practitioners and users. Reciprocally, if contact times have been arranged, it is essential that they should be honoured.

Quality of contact
This is the degree of openness and honesty which can be achieved, together with the degree of mutuality, so that each practitioner is really listening to the other and sharing information fully. The success of any contact depends upon the degree of satisfaction obtained by the participants.

Availability of support systems

To meet the user's need successfully the practitioner needs opportunities to discuss caseloads, share possible solutions and to explore feelings. The source of support may vary. It may come from:

- the same narrow professional grouping;
- other members of the same profession or organisation;
- other community practitioners;
- an independent person.

Example

The primary care physiotherapist might use other members of the primary care team who undertand the task and the environment for emotional support, information and debate on appropriate community resources to tap, but turn to her own profession for support on therapeutic intervention decisions.

Access to resources

Resources include other services, other practitioners, equipment and information, the user himself, his immediate social circle and his environment.

Knowledge of how to access all these resources and how to use them appropriately is crucial to the quality and effectiveness of an intervention. It is also helpful to be aware of constraints which apply to these resources and to share with others the constraints which affect one's own practice.

There are resources which are not necessarily seen as part of the resource pool because of custom and local practice. For instance, a community physiotherapist might not consider day centres, group practice premises, community centres or recreation centres as potential areas for use in meeting need if the post has traditionally been solely domiciliary practice. These venues might prove ideal settings for advice sessions, health education or health promotion sessions, and these might allow better management of the workload to be introduced.

Teaching other practitioners in rest homes or clubs suitable activities, and sharing relevant knowledge, can enhance personal intervention, meet the users' needs more effectively than the limited time available to the professional, and add to the pool of people who can assist in similar circumstances in the future.

Status of the employing agency

Voluntary services, which have usually started in response to unmet user demand or to augment the state-provided services, are often more flexible, less hierarchical and freer of statutory obligation. They may be able to be more responsive to the extraordinary, 'nonconformist' or minority need.

Example

A 66-year-old woman could be totally independent if she could walk as far as her local shops. She enquired for assistance in obtaining a pavement scooter. She did not qualify for mobility allowance, being over age, but a charity organisation linked with her previous employment was prepared to contribute part of the cost. Her local Good Neighbours group, for which she did some voluntary work, decided that they were willing to coordinate an appeal on her behalf provided that the Aids and Equipment Centre for their area would advise on the most appropriate vehicle.

Parameters for the user

In the same way that there are parameters on the practitioner there are similar ones placed upon the user:

- Changes in status, often linked with the reason that assistance is sought.
- Previous experience or hearsay evidence of the social services overall or of the one from which help is sought.
- Life experience which influences attitudes towards the providers, the interpretation of the problem, the understanding of it, and reactions to it, and interactions with other people be they service practitioners, family or friends.
- Expectations of the likely outcome of intervention, together with those of people in contact with the user.
- Communication between practitioners and user. Practitioners need to ensure that language has common meaning and jargon is avoided so that there is mutual understanding. If the command of the common language limits understanding and the quality of the contact it is better to work through an appropriate interpreter.
- Access to other support or help is made possible by the initial contact practitioner having the appropriate information to share or access to other services.

Example

The working manager of his own business had a stroke which meant that he was unable to work. He lost the social status which his business had given him as well as declining economic status. Prior to his stroke he had not needed to use any of the Social Services or Social Benefits. His only previous encounter had been when a staff member's son had a serious road accident, leaving him with permanent disability. This had resulted in the home needing adaptations and assessment for various benefits. The erstwhile manager recalled the apparent hassle and difficulties which this staff member had related, and his apparent dislike of some of the many people who had been involved. He was very apprehensive about how his own needs would be met, defensive of his old status, and yet unsure of how he would cope in his vulnerable position.

The first practitioner he encountered respected his former status and took time to explain procedures to him, ensuring that he understood the terms and implications of them by avoiding using jargon words without explaining their meaning.

He was further reassured about other people being involved in his misfortune by the practitioner relating referrals to his previous experience as a manager where he used the best person for the job. This abated his apprehensiveness as it gave him the essential background for him to be involved in reordering his life and to enable him to feel in control again.

Finance

Some key influences on finance are:

Political priorities

At national level the share of the financial resources allocated to the social services depends upon the political priorities of the government. At local level finance allocated may be even more dependent upon political priorities as individual council members may have special interests in or personal priorities between the different sectors of the statutory services.

Personality

The personality of the person championing a service or cause can influence the distribution of finance. This can lead to unequal distribution, particularly when comparing provision between authorities or the funds raised by collectors for the same cause.

Appeal of the cause

A cause or user group which has more general appeal to potential financers tends to gain a larger share of the available finance. Children's charities and voluntary services hold more appeal than those for elderly people.

Wealth

Where a community has a relatively high number of moneyed retired people, who are usually healthier and longer living than their working class counterparts, they become fundraisers and/or volunteers for what they perceive as worthy causes.

Local government policies

The interpretation of national government policy and the statutory requirements will be influenced by local politics, current social provision and local need.

Money for elderly social care may be channelled to support the home carers' service rather than a day centre and transport to it. Similarly, money allocated in health to improving elderly care may be devoted to day hospital facilities or establishing a travelling unit and additional community staff.

Within education the resources allocated for special needs will be allocated relative to the current provision in different schools and the number of children with special needs in those schools.

Local grants to voluntary organisations may be targeted differently from one year to another depending on particular local need and issues, and any particular demands placed on certain organisations by the support given to local authorities in meeting their statutory obligations.

Local population structure

Some factors which can influence services provision and delivery and also impinge on each other are:

The age population structure
The highest users of caring services are the elderly and families with children under three. Any locality with above national averages in these age groups will need to consider the implications for its care provision.

Cultural mix
In areas where there are mixed cultures and fairly large ethnic minority groups local authorities have to consider the different use made of services, together with the ways in which services are acceptable to the different groups, whilst being seen to be fair to all residents.

The health status
There may be local epidemiological factors, possibly from the effects of local industries, past or present, or from population stasis in the past causing close intermarriage and recessive genetic effects to come to the fore.

The social class mix
This influences need, demand, local support, and the recruitment pool available for different services.

The stability of the population
Where there is a fairly static population there is more likely to be a close-knit community with local family and neighbourhood support. In areas with constantly changing residents this support tends to be lacking.

Example

In a locality where 50% of the population are retired middle class there is likely to be greater demand for home care assistance, disability aids and minor home adaptations. There could also be greater demand for day centres, suitable transport, sheltered housing, suitable recreational and social facilities and meals on wheels. It could be difficult to find sufficient people to staff the home care services assessed as needed, particularly as some of this group, although more able, may well be competing in the restricted local employment pool by employing their own help. There may well be a greater than usual pool of volunteers, though their offers of assistance may not meet local need and be devoted to national interests.

Local topography

The geography, such as mountains, hills and rivers; the geology, such as the underlying rock strata and soil types; and features such as marshes, heaths, forests and other land use, all affect the distribution of settlements and the communication routes between them.

Example

In South Wales where coal was found, the deep coal pits were developed as industry's demand outstripped the supply from surface and drift mines. Workers needed to be housed within walking distance of the pit heads. With the bleakness and barrenness of the mountains, and the need for water and supplies, homes tended to be built in the narrow valleys. Roads could not be built from one valley head to another as there were few natural passes so communication followed the river courses.

Small health, educational and social facilities may be sited in these villages and towns, but major facilities to serve the area may be difficult to site and involve long journeys to reach, although not distant as the crow flies.

Housing

The type of housing, the density and the local policy for renewal, replacement or development all influence services. The number of dwellings in multiple occupancy in a locality, and the change in use of housing stock also have an effect.

The local interpretation of government policies for housing renewal may lead to demolition and rebuilding or to efforts to restore and improve the quality of the existing dwellings. There may be efforts to keep the local community together, or rehousing elsewhere take place and a new community arise.

Development may be new estates where there can be a bias of social class or age, or infilling which can also alter the age and social structure of a locality. In some areas development is not allowed. This leads to families having to move away from their roots against their wills with less ease of immediate family support when needed.

Housing usage can alter. In an area where there has been a number of large family homes, some may be redeveloped for multiple occupancy, which can be a change of use to rest home, sheltered housing or student accommodation. Others may be demolished for flats to be built or a new estate of some kind. All increase the density of population which change service provision and need. Conversely density can be reduced by small adjoining cottages being converted into one larger family dwelling. The design of a house and the access to it affects the need for adaptation or rehousing if someone living in it becomes disabled. A small terrace house with a small back yard and a passage step to the kitchen limits the life for a wheelchair user to one room. A similar one with a wider passage and enough space to build a downstairs toilet and shower may be adaptable.

Some Local Authorities use hostels for homeless people whilst others might use short-life housing for temporary accommodation or bed and breakfast accommodation. This can cause difficulties for continuing health and social care, and education where children are involved. Redevelopment plans can alter the character of an area and the desirability of living there, changing the population mix. Once development is complete the desirability can alter again and new people of a different background settle.

Transport systems

If local transport links directly with facilities and key shopping areas, and is frequent, the elderly and less able are less dependent upon community and family goodwill than those with poor transport and those without cars. Changes in transport which reduce ease of access can socially disadvantage the less active and carless. It can change the use of services.

Example

An over-sixties club near a shopping precinct had a high membership, but when a bus route was withdrawn as it was not used regularly enough club membership was halved. Those unable to reach the venue found their social focus had gone, leaving them socially isolated and depressed, as well as altering where, when and how they did their shopping. A need emerged for some replacement transport or a similar club very locally and, for some, assistance with weekly shopping.

A change in the design of the local buses or trains can also alter use depending on how easy the vehicles are to board and leave and whether there is anyone available to assist should help be needed.

For the service provider there is likely to be more need for home or very local services where transport is poor or there is some distance to transport stops.

Patterns of traffic flow, such as density of traffic at different times of day, one-way systems, use of alternative routes and changes to road systems also need consideration by the service provider. A distance of a mile in peak times can take up to 10 minutes, but only 2 or 3 minutes at quiet times. A road closure to stop traffic taking a short cut through a residential area may involve replanning routes and appointment schedules.

Population expectation

Expectation of services is affected by social class and previous experience. Media coverage can alter expectations, either by heightening demand for a service or casting doubt upon the value of a current provision. The debate over the Peto method of treatment for children with cerebral palsy is a prime example. The media can also direct demand away from statutory provision towards voluntary or private provision.

Local employment

The nature of employment has major implications upon the health and social wellbeing of a community as well as its economic viability. Some communities are virtually dependent upon one major employer. Any change in its employment policy has a knock-on effect on other businesses and their employees. The input of local social services will be affected by that major industry's welfare policies and provisions. High employment and plenty of employment opportunities enhances social and health wellbeing. Unemployment produces stress amongst the unemployed and their families, which in turn affects their healthy functioning in all aspects of life and is likely to increase need for social services.

Services' personnel

The services are affected by the personnels':

- qualifications;
- level of competence;
- previous experience;
- attitudes;
- opportunities for personal development;
- recruitment.

Well qualified enthusiastic staff who show a high level of competence tend to have positive attitudes to their work. These in turn attract new staff whose skills are extended by example as well as by specific educational opportunities being made available to all levels of staff.

Exercises

1. Look at your own locality and analyse the effects of these parameters upon it.
2. Within your own organisation discover:

   - how information is collected on local need;
   - by what process resources are allocated to meet those needs;
   - how the use of resources is monitored.

3. Find out the local machinery that ensures coordination of services.

Putting community care into practice

The practitioner's management of self

Any practitioner needs to have a system to be efficient and make best use of the working day. The main framework is established by the organisation employing the practitioner, but within this framework each practitioner will have an individual daily work schedule. For the community practitioner providing a service there are a number of variables which will need to be taken into account when planning work to ensure that the day is used wisely and fits into the working hours. These are as follows.

User accessibility for contact

Some users have other responsibilities, care needs or demands for contact time placed upon them which might take priority. This can limit the time available for a practitioner to meet with the user, or, if certain services are only available at certain times, limits the choice of service provision that can be made for that user.

> ***Example***
>
> Mr D. attends the Travelling Day Centre on Tuesdays for social contact, lunch, bathing and other personal needs. His wife has a regular commitment which she is able to meet on Tuesdays. The therapist thought the best way of helping with his arthritic condition was for him to join the arthritic group, but this only meets on Tuesdays. A different solution was found.

Travel factors

The practitioner is expected to use the shortest or most economical means of travel. Road travel can be affected by:

Time of day
Some routes are very congested at particular times of day. A slightly longer route may reduce travel time and prove more economical in the long run for paid practitioners when the busy time of day cannot be avoided in the day schedule.

The weekday
Street markets or other special events can exclude a route. Work schedules need planning to avoid the affected areas as much as possible on those days. Workers in tourist and holiday areas find that the visitors' routes can mean a different pattern of routes and work schedules at different times of the year.

One-way systems
Routes which take note of these should be planned. It may be

quicker to park a car and walk rather than taking a long detour around a circuit.

Diversions

As local press notices and bill boards give details in advance of planned diversions and road closures it is worthwhile keeping a watch for them.

Parking

In some areas this can be so difficult that using public transport, cycling, or walking may be a more efficient use of time and money, as well as keeping the worker fit.

Even where special service and employment discs are displayed they do not allow exemption from parking regulations. Getting to know local traffic wardens and seeking their assistance can be worthwhile for practitioners regularly in a locality.

Arrangements might be possible with service users if requested at the time of arranging a visit, or with other services with parking in the area.

Weather

Snow, ice, hail, fog, gales and heavy rain make travel hazardous. More time should be allowed for travel in the winter. If road conditions are very bad personal safety may override user needs. It may be wiser not to venture out but to telephone users to see if there is any advice that can help until it is possible to visit.

Communication systems

Communication is essential for coordinated community care, both between the various community services and any other services which have been used or may be of value to the user and carers. Community practitioners, by the very nature of their work, are not at one point of contact during the working day. Effective systems need to be established so that time is not wasted whilst practitioners are trying to contact each other.

Letters, which take time to write, or special forms, can be used but may be slow, particularly when a response is required. A mobile phone, Ansaphone or message clerk can help with contact. One solution is for the practitioner to regularly be at a definite place at a fixed time of the day so that other practitioners can call there. For preference this would be during standard rate telephone time but this is not always possible or practicable. If a message has been left for another practitioner to call between certain times these arrangements should be honoured. The other practitioner may have had to make special arrangements to make contact. If another person's phone is used to make calls, the call should be timed and payment made. Most people underestimate the duration of calls, especially when they are doing most of the talking!

Administrative needs

Various information and data will need to be recorded. How this is done will depend upon the service organisation's requirements, but even if clerical support is provided the community practitioner will require time:

- to arrange appointments;
- to complete records;
- to prepare letters, reports and training material;
- to arrange equipment supply and delivery;
- to attend meetings;
- for data collection and analysis;
- for evaluation and forward planning.

Personal support needs

1. One of the most important functions of support is to diminish inappropriate guilt feelings which sap morale and efficiency. When a person is working in a caring service in isolation from other practitioners the demands placed upon them can seem overwhelming at times. They should not feel guilty in setting aside time for their own emotional support. Without this other users may receive a poor quality service from a drained and indecisive practitioner.

Example

Some community practitioners feel that they are 'wasting time' when they are not actually with a service user, even when they are aware that administration and communication are part of their work. Surveys have shown that although distributed in different ways during the working day, the length of time spent on such duties remains fairly constant, regardless of the setting in which a person works. They may also feel guilty about the time spent in activity not specific to their own profession or task, even when they realise that this activity enhances the particular intervention.

Time to reflect upon one's work, seek professional stimulation and to keep up to date with relevant developments is also necessary if the worker is to remain effective in intervention.

2. Personal safety system should be observed. There are some locations and some homes where it is inadvisable to venture alone. It may be necessary to go at the same time as another practitioner. If you are aware of any place which falls into this category all other practitioners who might be involved should be warned of the circumstances to protect them.

There are also areas where it is considered unsafe to be after dark, so care should be taken to complete visits with time in hand before dusk. All practitioners should ensure that their whereabouts are known, which is most easily done by leaving a copy of the day's visit locations with phone numbers where possible at the contact base. This is also helpful if a late message comes in to cancel a visit or there is urgent need to contact the practitioner.

3. A system to cope with delays should be decided. If the practitioner has both small change and a phone card it should be possible to either phone a person direct, or if a person is at base, contact there and ask for other calls to be made. Should a visit be delayed where there is no phone, apology is the only recourse.

4. It is helpful when making appointments to try to leave leeway in times, by arranging that you will call between certain times. Most users appreciate that it is not possible to accurately predict the duration of visits or what travel conditions will be like.

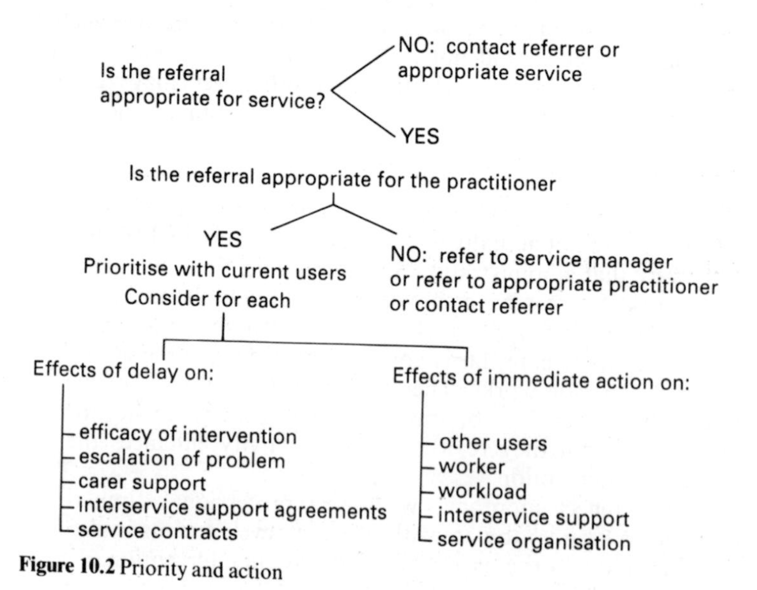

Figure 10.2 Priority and action

Where possible gaps should be left between some appointments to allow for urgent visits or for the occasional hold up. There is always either administration or self-education that can be carried out should those gaps not be filled, or a liaison contact with other workers that can be made.

Priorities of user need

With any service decisions have to be taken all the time on which users should be included or excluded if the service is to cope with the demands placed upon it. This also applies to the practitioner and to the organisation of the daily work schedules.

A method of deciding priority and action is to consider the method shown in Figure 10.2:

Example

The physiotherapist finds that the new referrals for the day are for

- an acute chest condition;
- urgent replacement of a broken walking frame;
- an urgent request to assist a man who cannot get to the toilet;
- man had stroke yesterday at breakfast time, right hemiplegia, nurse visiting today;
- mobility trolley for kitchen use – disabled man just widowed.

The mobility trolley is supplied by the Social Services occupational therapist. The referral is passed across and the referrer informed. The other referrals are deemed appropriate but further information is sought about the man who cannot get to the toilet. It is found that he has acute back pain and has been advised to rest in bed. A phone call to order a commode from short-term loan is advised and arrangement made to see the man in the next few days. A phone call to the frame user elicits the type and size, and the problem with the present frame. A replacement is ordered by phone so that it can be delivered at the group practice by lunch time for the physiotherapist to take out that afternoon. This leaves the acute chest patient, whose problem is likely to escalate if intervention is delayed, and the stroke patient. The service agreements are that acute chests will be seen the same day as referral and strokes within 48 hours of onset. As the nurse is visiting, some support will be given to the carer.

Exercise

Preferably in a group

The day's appointments so far are:

8.30–9.00 Base office – administration, communication time. The office is 4 minutes' drive to southeast of work locality edge.
9.15–10.15 Case conference at patient's house – south in patch.
11.15 Second visit, multiple sclerosis patient – east in patch.
12.15 Group practice meeting over lunch – west in patch.
1.30 First visit, osteoarthritic patient (no phone) – west in patch.
2.30 Final check on poor mobility patient – west side of central.
Check visit chronic bronchitis patient on self management programme – north side of central.
3.20 Check visit to rheumatoid arthritic re new splints and home management (son there 3.00–4.15) – north in patch.
4.30 Base office – administrative, communication time (return call expected).
5.00 Finish work – friends due at 7.00 for dinner.

The new patients mentioned in the example have to be fitted into this schedule.

The acute chest patient lives in the extreme south-west of the patch, which will mean at least 10 minutes' travel from the nearest locations, and it takes you 20 minutes to go from north to south of your patch, and 25 minutes east to west. The stroke patient lives east central and the replacement frame goes to a south central resident.

Consider how you can organise the day.

Management of the problem

A helpful approach towards arranging successful community care is to use a problem-orientated approach towards resolution.

To manage any problem it is essential to:

- recognise the reason given for the approach for help;

- identify the cause of the problem so that a plan of intervention to resolve or diminish that problem can be made;
- recognise the strengths and weaknesses of the user, his personal contacts and his environment.

To achieve this in the community setting, and particularly when community care is to take place in the user's home, the aspects to be considered are:

- physical, psychological, social and environmental;
- the interactions between the user, his family and/or current carers and the user's wider social circle.

This will allow the context of the problem to be identified, together with the key points for intervention.

The delivery of care

Success is achieved in community based care when there is *commitment, sharing* and *enabling* in *partnership*.

Throughout the delivery of care this should always be at the forefront of the practitioner's mind.

The delivery of care in the community can take place either in the user's home, at a services facility such as in a group practice, health centre, school or day centre, or in a communal facility, such as a recreation centre or social centre.

Whichever setting is the focal point the same basic process can be followed for the individual, although variations will occur in how the care is delivered.

Setting the scene

This starts with the decision that the user should be included in the workload and offered the service.

The practitioner will gather relevant background information, whether direct from the user or from the referrer, related to:

- the problem itself;
- any action already taken by other agencies which will impinge on the practitioner's intervention;
- the user – any detail that might impinge on the problem and its resolution, e.g. employment, responsibilities, daily routine, pets;
- the family circle when intervention is likely to involve the members in any way;

- the home – an overview, its location and access if care in the home is to take place.

This sets the scene and begins to give the context of the problem together with the possible intervention. It also allows the priority of this user's need to be assessed in relation to the rest of the practitioner's caseload, and, where there is choice on the location of the intervention, an appropriate choice of venue to be made for the initial contact.

Collecting information

When with the user the sources of information are:

- verbal, which includes the way and tone in which things are said, the pauses, or lack of them, and what is left unsaid;
- non-verbal, which includes the body language, eye contact etc.
- environmental, which includes the physical social and psychological aspects.

In a family or caring situation the same level of observation is required of the others present. They are of equal importance to the success or failure of any intervention. Because people operate within the family and social systems it is impossible to view their problems in isolation from the people involved. One-dimensional assessments which ignore the social setting will often prove misleading.

Example

Mrs T. lived in sheltered housing. She stated that she got on well with the other residents but rarely joined in the coffee mornings and other group events as she had always been a 'loner', preferring to stay at home making craft items for charities.

She had been referred as increased shoulder and knee pain, with reduced mobility from generalised arthritis. There were no clinical signs to account for her altered symptoms, and her movements were quite spry. She was concerned that she was finding it difficult to get her shopping and was thinking of getting a pavement scooter, but had been told by the warden that she would not be able to keep it in the corridor alcove outside her flat.

When leaving, the therapist met other residents known to her as they left the coffee morning. They guessed whom she had been visiting and commiserated with the therapist, saying what a 'difficult' lady she was. She had fallen out with nearly all of them and was always arguing with the warden. Her latest contretemps had resulted in them all having to move items kept in the space under the stairs, even those allowed by the Fire Officer.

Exercise

What weight would you give to information gathered in this way? How does it alter your perception? How would you use this information in your work with Mrs T.?

Listen to the carers

Carers often have valuable observations, as well as feelings and opinions, to contribute to the care programme. They will notice *how* people perform, and the effects of the environment both on the individual as well as on themselves.

Example

Mrs T. was caring for her son K., who had been discharged from the neurosurgical unit following a major blockage of his valve draining and controlling his hydrocephalus. He was sent home after intensive rehabilitation with considerable extensor spasm, but able to stand and walk with assistance, using a full length caliper on his left leg to control it. Mr and Mrs T. had to assist with his personal needs.

The community physiotherapist had been asked to visit to ensure that K.'s parents were coping with the handling and his maintenance exercises. On the therapist's third visit, Mrs T. remarked that she had accidentally given K. a cold shower that morning. K. remarked that it was 'typical of Mum – didn't listen to my protest', but Mrs T. had noticed that he was more relaxed and easier to dress.

Although it was 2 hours later, the therapist also found there was less muscle spasm. Ice had been tried before but found not of benefit, but the cold water had obviously helped. K. felt himself that it would be worth 'suffering' again to see if this was not just a 'one-off' result. The physiotherapist called 2 days later and found that the cold shower was having a general relaxing effect. She decided that the really tight left leg muscles might benefit from wrapping in an iced towel during the afternoon to assist and overcome the increased spasm that occurred when he started tiring.

Without the observation the therapist would probably not have tried ice again at this stage in light of the previous rehabilitation record.

Problem analysis

When the practitioner is sifting the information gathered a matter of primary import will be whether the presenting problem is the symptom or the cause.

Although each community practitioner has specific areas of expertise their observations will often lead to a wider understanding of the problem than is strictly within their brief. This should not be ignored since effective intervention will often require more than one practitioner's input. Just treating the referred problem will sometimes only address the symptom and not the underlying cause of the difficulty, which, if left, will only erupt again when stress is high.

Even with structure to the information gathering, it is common to find that information is jumbled. The key issues will need to be identified. It can be helpful to list key words reflecting the immediate concerns where there seem to be a large number of problem areas or information seems confusing. This:

- clarifies the situation by showing which issues might be remedied;
- gives opportunity to order the problems into the short and long term;
- enables a checklist to be agreed with the user before any action plan is made.

Planning resolution

Each community practitioner will need to identify:

- what would be their specific intervention, if any;
- what other intervention would be desirable;
- what intervention would be possible.

Adding to the key word list, two further columns noting resources and constraints will help identify possible interventions and enable a possible action plan to be drawn up which can then be discussed with the service user.

Action plan

The plan is drawn up in partnership with the user, and, where relevant, with other carers. It is important that there is:

- mutual agreement and understanding of the problem(s);
- possible intervention(s) and the implications are explained and understood by those who are likely to be affected;
- the service user is able to express their views and come to informed decisions about acceptance of the suggestions.

It may not be appropriate to tackle everything at once where there are several matters requiring attention. The practitioner will need to judge the most appropriate starting point, especially when identifying problems. The user may not wish to share information or identify any issues which do not appear to have a direct bearing on the reason for the practitioner being present. This privacy should be respected.

As the action plan is being drawn up short term and long term outcome goals should be identified so that the user knows what is expected, and so that the practitioner has a checklist to enable the plan to be monitored and adapted as required.

Further action

This will depend upon the initial action but will normally include:

- a review of the previous meeting;
- a check on the effect of that intervention;
- consideration of how the user has complied with points of the plan;
- evaluating the impact of the intervention, i.e. whether there have been any difficulties or misunderstandings caused by the intervention;
- identification of any new issues which affect the plan;
- adjustments made to the long-term goals if necessary;
- the setting of new short-term goals;
- monitoring of overall progress.

It may well be that new issues are introduced that influence the way forward. It is incumbent on the practitioner to stay open to the situation and to deal with these issues as they arise. If the issue is one for which nothing can be done, it should be acknowledged as such in an appropriate manner.

Terminating contact

It is desirable that the user should feel that a satisfactory result has been obtained, although this is not always possible. It can sometimes be difficult to withdraw but if the long-term and short-term goals have been addressed the user will be aware of the likely withdrawal of the practitioner. There are always some users who find new 'problems' or reasons why contact should be continued. In these instances, where the practitioner is sure that all that can be achieved has been and the user has understood the outcome of the intervention, assertiveness needs to come to the fore.

Where a particular visit is difficult to terminate, it is often helpful for the practitioner to state on arrival how long there is for the visit, and when this time is nearly up to remind the user of it, whilst making sure that the next visit is arranged with sufficient time to cover mutual need. This is important if some key issue is brought up as the practitioner is leaving, since the user may have found it difficult to raise the issue and needs to feel that it has value. The appointment should be arranged with the intention of looking at the issue.

Example case study

Setting the scene

Widowed Mrs D., who lived in a terrace house, was referred to the physiotherapist in late November with neck and shoulder pain which had got worse in the past few weeks. It was noted that she was an old polio who had had neck problems some years ago and who also suffered from bronchial asthma. This had also been more troublesome of late, so a home visit was being requested, but with a note to phone first. The current medication was listed.

Using the service delivery chart (Figure 10.2, p. 280), it was felt the referral was acceptable and a home visit would be made. This was arranged.

Collecting information

On arrival it was noted that she lived about 100 yards on a slight gradient down from a corner shop which had notices 'under new management' on the window. Her 9 foot deep front garden was level and paved, with two feature shrubs either side of the window bay. The house exterior was well maintained. The windows were polished with fresh net curtains behind the lower sashes. The brass letter-box, knocker and doorstep edge shone. When the physiotherapist knocked on the door, Mrs D. peeped from behind a net curtain. On coming to the door one of two security locks was opened and she checked who was there before releasing the door chain.

In the passage there was a hallstand with two men's coats, a cap and her 'errand' coat, two long walking sticks and some umbrellas. The passage runner was fixed down, with the exposed lino highly polished. The physiotherapist was taken into the front room and the gas fire lit. Several photos stood on the sideboard, the most prominent being a portrait of a young soldier taken in the Second World War.

After introductions, Mrs D. launched into a catalogue of her medical problems, but interspersed with these was how much she missed her husband. He had helped her move things and massaged her neck and shoulders for her when they ached as her polio had left her with weak shoulders and upper arms. Whilst relating this her voice was plaintive and she was close to tears, wringing her hands.

She then apologised, saying 'I really shouldn't grumble as lots of people are worse off than me, but it's so nice to see a sympathetic face. I haven't anyone to talk to now as my neighbours of 25 years moved to live near their son 2 months ago – I do miss them – and now the corner shop family have gone too. I think I must be one of the few old residents left – so many places have changed hands and everyone goes out to work now.'

A gentle enquiry revealed that her husband had died just a year ago. Her only daughter was happily married, living in Canada with her two children. There had been talk of her joining them but she did not want to leave her home and memories yet. She also thought that their lifestyle was so different that she would not feel at home. She did not want to impose on them as they had their own lives to lead. She also wondered how the cold air would affect her chest, but she did wish she could visit, although she hated flying and travelling on her own.

When the therapist asked about how she slept, and with what pillows, she was taken upstairs. The late Mr D.'s personal belongings were still much in evidence – his dressing gown still hung on the door, and his book and spectacles were by the bed. There were some sleeping pills on the dressing table but she said she did not take them, even though she did not sleep as well as she used to do. She kept busy cleaning and polishing because she found if she kept occupied the day didn't seem so long and she slept better at night.

Problem analysis

From the information provided by the verbal and non-verbal behaviour, it was possible to gain an insight into this lady's inner world. Mrs D.'s true problem was her unresolved grief for her husband and the other lesser bereavements of losing a valued part of her social network. Her asthma, shoulder and neck pain were worsened by her distress and her sense of isolation which left her feeling very vulnerable. Her need to keep busy was also affecting her physically by her choice of a familiar activity.

Exercise

- Identify the case material which has led to this statement of 'vulnerability'.
- Before reading on, jot down the key words for likely intervention and add your list of resources and constraints.

Planning resolution

The physiotherapist had jotted down some key words as she was listening to Mrs D. and whilst she was carrying out her clinical assessment. They then talked together and agreed that the key issues were as listed. The therapist also noted possible resources and likely constraints.

Problem	*Resources*	*Constraints*
Grief	Counselling, CRUSE*	May need transport
Isolation/ loneliness	Over 60's club, Good neighbour scheme, Voluntary visitors, CHA† club (give/receive help), Polio Fellowship Independence; practicality	Smokey atmosphere Wary of strangers Fear of losing 'face' Cold aggravates chest
Neck/shoulder pain	Heat, exercises, relaxtion	Old polio Houseproud Way of doing things Posture
Asthma	Breathing exercises, exercise tolerance programme, asthmatic group, check use of inhaler	Tried them before! Previous experience
Need of daughter/ confidant	Travel club; regular mail; telephone; good relationship with son-in-law Friendliness; pleasant	Fear of solo travel No wish to impose

* CRUSE: The National Organisation for the Widowed and their Children.
† CHA: The Chest and Heart Association.

It will be noted that independence appears as a resource and a constraint. Listing helps to decide a method of approach which takes this into consideration.

Exercise

Compare your list with this. Where there are differences is it because you are from a different background (not a physiotherapist) or you have missed a clue, or noticed other points?

Action plan

The action plan drawn up in discussion with Mrs D. was:

- Means of heat application to her neck and shoulders to relieve pain.
- Relaxation via contrast muscle tension and deep breathing.
- Shoulder girdle and neck exercises to relax muscle tension and improve mobility and pain-free range of movement.
- Reduce the present method of polishing and cleaning which aggravated her neck/shoulder pain but start to look at alternative ways which would assist in maintaining or building up strength in her weaker polio-affected muscles with the occupational therapist.
- Arrange for her to attend the physiotherapy department so that a baseline of her chest function could be obtained.
- Consider whether some social contact source would be beneficial.
- See following week.

Short-term goals for Mrs D. were:

- to reduce her shoulder/neck pain by compliance with the physiotherapy programme;
- not to do heavy work for the coming week;
- to think back to what her cleaning system had been when she had no pain problems;
- to go for a short walk each day, weather permitting, possibly to the shop;
- to decide whether to take up some of the 'social' options.

The walk was set to maintain her general exercise tolerance and with the hope that she would see someone else at some time each day. The request to outline her 'pain-free' cleaning system was to gain some knowledge of her previous activity level and ability, so that appropriate long-term goals could be set.

Mrs D. was expecting physiotherapy advice for her neck/shoulder problem, so it was an appropriate starting point for the physiotherapist. This plan recognises the physical problems and treats the symptoms, whilst tackling the underlying causes of it. It also acknowledges her standards of housekeeping and her need for a social outlet. There is credibility and an acceptable reason for her to go out where she would meet other people aware of her presenting problem.

When considering how she could establish social contact it was suggested that she might wish to assist others less able than herself in some way, as well as suggesting joining a local lunch club or interest group. The suggestion of a visitor was not made as it was thought that if Mrs D. could be encouraged to go out a little this would be of more benefit.

From this it can be seen that the long-term goal was to re-establish Mrs D.'s social life, and enable her to live without aggravating her physical weakness, thus improving her quality of life.

After the visit contact was made with the occupational therapist and the respiratory physiotherapist, and arrangements made for them to see Mrs D. on the same visit to the rehabilitation department.

Further action

On arriving the next week the physiotherapist found Mrs D. looking less tense and very welcoming. Mrs D. had found using a warm hot water bottle across her shoulders whilst sitting back in her chair very comforting. She had found that she could relax better if she practised half an hour after using her asthma inhaler and after she had done her mobilising exercises. She had not done any unnecessary heavy tasks – she said doing her exercises had occupied her time! She felt a lot easier and on working out her old cleaning routine realised just how much she had been doing to fill her time.

She was now looking forward to her visit to the hospital department to see the occupational therapist. She still wasn't too sure that it would be worth the time of the chest physiotherapist because she had been told several times that she would have to live with her chest problem. She was not sure how she would get there if the weather was bad, as she found waiting for the change of buses made her very wheezy and achey.

She had thought about social groups. If there was somewhere she could be useful she might like that, and she wouldn't mind joining a lunch club, so long as they weren't full of 'funny' people, and she could get there. She found it had helped her being able to talk last week too, so if CRUSE people were like the therapist she would give it a try. Her daughter had written a long letter and she told the therapist a little of her news.

The physiotherapist suggested she contact her surgery about getting to hospital as, if she did not qualify for hospital transport, they would be able to arrange for the local Care group to help. Since she had a telephone she might find that the Care group would like her help later on.

Her exercises and relaxation technique were checked and modified, with some minor corrections being made. Mrs D. felt a sense of achievement from the therapist being pleased with her progress and the way she had done her exercises.

Mrs D. agreed not to 'go mad' again over the housework. A way of coping with the essential heavier work was discussed. If she found what she did in a day aggravated her shoulders she would ease off and stay with the little less strenuous for a day or so before trying again.

The CRUSE contact was given to Mrs D. along with that of the voluntary help coordinator. Mrs D. wanted the therapist to make contact for her but she was encouraged to do this herself. She rang the CRUSE contact before the therapist left and found it not as difficult to do as she had thought. The therapist would be contacting the local lunch club and asking the organiser to get in touch with Mrs D. since self-referral was unusual.

Mrs D. was very apologetic that she had not been out for a short walk each day, but it had been wet and windy twice, and this aggravated her chest. The therapist said she had not expected her to go out on bad days, but was pleased she had gone along to the shop on the other days. On being asked how she found the new people there, Mrs D. said they were very pleasant though young, and she hoped they would be able to make a go of the shop. They had two children of about 6 and 7, who reminded her of her grandchildren. They were certainly working hard and had a big Christmas display. Since she would be on her own this year she was going to treat Christmas as an ordinary day, but no doubt she 'would croak along with the carols on TV and radio', as she had always done. Just as the therapist thought Mrs D. was leaving the subject, Mrs D. remarked that she hoped her family would understand why she hadn't been able to send lots of presents as they usually had but it wasn't easy to manage just on her pension with the house to keep up as well. Her husband had always done the repairs and looked after the house bills. She hadn't realised how much work cost until she had to pay this past week for her back window to be repaired.

The physiotherapist thought that there might be other benefits she could claim, but Mrs D. responded that they had always managed and paid their way without charity so she wasn't starting now. It was pointed out that her husband had paid his national insurance so it was not charity but a right if she qualified for other benefits, in the same way as her state pension. Would she like the benefits and rights adviser, who was very discreet, to meet her to see whether she was entitled to any more? Mrs D. replied that if her Bill had paid towards these other benefits then he would want her to have them so perhaps it would be a good idea. That day the therapist made contact with the benefits adviser who asked that Mrs D. should phone her to arrange an appointment. The message was passed on for Mrs D. to decide upon making contact.

Exercise

Identify the further action stages. Were the physiotherapist's responses always appropriate? Have you noted any other of Mrs D.'s personal resources?

Next visit

At this visit the results of her time with the respiratory physiotherapist were discussed and the slight modification to her previous routine checked. Mrs D. had been surprised that the physiotherapist had contacted her GP about her inhalers, but she found that her GP had been expecting to hear following the discussion of the community physiotherapist's action plan. She felt less tight in her chest as a result of the altered routine, although she really had not thought that she would.

She had found the occupational therapist very helpful with some longstanding difficulties from her polio as well as suggesting ways she could cope with the heavier tasks without aggravating her shoulders and neck. She wished she had met an OT years ago.

Her shoulder/neck pain had almost gone. A check was made that Mrs D. understood what to do to prevent recurrence, and should one happen, what to do to help herself. Directions were written down in her words, and the use of each part of her programme checked through with her. She had been visited by a CRUSE counsellor and also been taken to a meeting. She had nearly called the visit off because she had worried that she might let herself down in front of strangers, but she had found everyone friendly and understanding.

The benefits adviser had been and helped her fill in some forms, and she was also having a visit from a 'staying put' scheme worker about her house maintenance.

The local stroke club wanted someone to help with refreshments and to help those with poor speech. She could be picked up if the weather was bad too. She had gone for the first time the day before and found she had enjoyed it; she had met a lady she hadn't seen for 15 years who used to live nearby too. The lunch club organiser had been in touch but she didn't feel it right to start with the Christmas dinner. They had agreed that they would decide in the New Year whether she would go. She added that she wouldn't have so much time to fill with polishing now so didn't think she was likely to get in such a bad way again – 'and I know what to do if I do happen to hit a bad patch'.

She then asked what the therapist was doing for Christmas. The therapist realised that it was going to be a sad time for Mrs D., since she had spent last Christmas just after her husband's death with her old neighbours, but she shared the plans for the quiet family celebration she was anticipating. Mrs D. then told her that the people at the shop had asked her if she would like to go along to share their Christmas dinner. She hadn't liked to accept at first, but they had been so nice, saying that they had lost her mother recently, which was how they'd come to the shop, and would be on their own, missing her. Since she wouldn't have her family with her that perhaps they could help each other by filling each others' gap. Her daughter had booked a phone call for Christmas Eve and her old neighbours had invited her too. Their son was going to collect her on Christmas evening and she was staying over for two nights, the first time she had been away since her husband died. She really felt that she had something to live for and to look forward to the New Year.

Exercise

- Check that all further action activities have been carried out.
- How is Mrs D. being prepared for terminating contact?

Terminating contact

Although the therapist was not arranging to call again she made sure that Mrs D. had the contact phone number she could call if she had any further problems, and reminded her that if her GP thought she needed any further help in the future he could arrange it too. Mrs D. was disappointed that the therapist was not coming again, but felt reassured that help was to hand through the contact number if she needed it as well as through her GP.

Exercises

- Analyse the different skills that were used in this interaction, apart from the direct physiotherapy intervention.
- This intervention took place just before Christmas. Do you think this made any difference to this intervention? If yes, in what way and why?

Chapter 11

Teaching in the community

Ann Compton and Mary Ashwin

Theory

Many community practitioners are unaware of how much of their day-to-day work involves teaching. Every community practitioner from time to time will be a teacher, and for some it is a major part of their role. Very often this role will be superimposed, or run alongside, other roles. For example, when working as a counsellor the practitioner has educative functions ranging from giving information to modelling new behaviours and demonstrating new styles of communication. The group practitioner, too, may be involved in attitude change, skills teaching and information giving. Family work has similar teaching aspects and community-based work abounds in both small and large group situations demanding a range of teaching strategies.

There are a number of tasks where teaching is the main skill involved. They include the following.

Information giving

This describes such activities as outlining a range of possible services, explaining the way in which particular equipment works, or how applications can be made for certain financial benefits or other resources. It is a way of widening the basis for choice.

Imparting knowledge to increase understanding

Information giving deals with gaps in information; imparting knowledge involves the practitioner in providing a new framework of understanding which will enable people to perceive their situation differently and manage it more appropriately. This might apply to teaching about a particular medical condition or the legal implications of certain behaviour. It often involves the introduction of concepts which may be quite foreign and which are frequently expressed in unfamiliar language.

Skills teaching

People need help to develop skills for a variety of reasons. These include:

Changes in physical and mental functioning
They may have become more or less able in some way, e.g. mobility may have improved or eyesight deteriorated.

Changes in the functioning of others
For example, carers may need new skills such as lifting in response to the condition of the person in their care.

Loss of skills
People may well need to relearn old skills which they have lost through social or physical circumstances, e.g. typing skill which had lain unused for some years but is now of value to use a computer.

Developmental requirements
Community practitioners may be involved in teaching new skills which will open up new opportunities. These might include skills concerned with personal hygiene, communication or the full exploitation of some new aid.

Environmental change
New environments make new demands and often people will find that they lack the skill required to manage these effectively. The move from institution into the community illustrates this type of need.

Awareness-raising work

The community practitioner will often be involved in this sort of learning both with individuals and/or groups. It is used in two main ways.

Self awareness work
Here people are provided with learning experiences which allow them to develop new understanding and insights both of themselves and their situations, providing a springboard for change and adjustment. An example might be a group of carers who are enabled to explore their reactions to their situations and discuss ways in which they might manage more effectively.

Issue awareness work

The techniques used will be similar to those for self awareness work, but since it is concerned with highlighting issues previously unexplored there will be greater emphasis on providing triggers to promote interest and concern, building on existing knowledge. Examples might be discussing the links between diet and fitness or stress and disease.

Attitude change

This differs from awareness work where the results are left open although the practitioner has a clear agenda. Many community practitioners have explicit briefs to work towards shifts in attitudes which will result in changes of behaviour. The nature of this change is already clearly formulated. Examples might include teaching on the effects of smoking on health or the practice of safe sex to prevent the spread of disease. At times this may present the practitioner with some ethical problems around freedom and choice.

Training and supervision

This will include all the preceding skills but is directed towards other helpers rather than service users. The distinction between training and supervision for the purposes of this chapter is that training is offered for the performance of specific tasks and supervision is concerned with overall professional performance and development. For example, volunteers may be trained to assist with mobility and stroke recovery, whilst each profession is increasingly offering supervision which includes management, especially quality assurance, teaching and support.

These various functions do not, in real life, come in neatly labelled divisions and many situations will contain elements from more than one of these categories. A person who has been severely injured in a road traffic accident and left with some serious permanent disability may require inputs of all the types described above. There are common elements which are crucial to effective teaching which apply across these categories and these will be addressed in the next section.

Exercise

Individually or in groups

- List the number of teaching situations in which you have been involved over the last 2 weeks.

- Divide them into the six categories given above.
- Discuss any special difficulties which you encounter in each of these teaching situations.

The ten commandments for community teachers

The following injunctions apply widely in situations which have some teaching component. They should be seen in the context of planned work as outlined in the chapter on assessment and programme planning.

1. Teaching must be a response to clearly identified needs

The common aim of all community practitioners is community health in its broadest sense. Because it is much easier to spot problems than define health we are tempted to become narrow and pathology focused in our work.

Educational needs should be defined positively in terms of opening up new opportunities and providing an additional range of choices. They are not met by providing ready-made solutions to tightly formulated problems. When we speak of clearly identified needs it is important that these are not seen merely in remedial terms for some malady located in the individual, family or social group. They should also be seen in terms of creating a social climate in which people arrive at their own definition of health and discover how to achieve it.

What is absolutely crucial is that the teacher has a vision of what they can contribute based on realistic assessment of their personal and professional competencies and of the people and situations with whom they interact.

2. What is taught must be seen to have relevance to the life of the learner

This is important for the motivation of the learner and therefore ultimately for the motivation of the teacher. Effective teaching has a sales component. Teachers need to convince their audience that they have something of value which is within the grasp of the listener even though its attainment may not be easy. The way in which information is conveyed is critical. Examples offered should be closely related to the lives of the listeners.

3. Learners must be engaged and involved in the learning experience

Before any learning can take place the interest of the hearer has to be caught and held. Acceptance and resignation are not useful ingredients in teaching situations, although they are very common in many situations which have been labelled as problematic. The belief that positive change is a real possibility and worth investment of time and energy is an essential prerequisite for both motivation and achievement.

4. The goals of each session must be identified and made known to the learner

Although there is an element of persuasion in teaching it is not a 'con job'. People need to know what is on offer, how it will be offered and what is expected from them if they are to participate fully. The preacher who said 'I tell them what I am going to tell them, then I tell them, then I tell them what I have told them' was no doubt successful. Inducing the right mental and emotional response is an important prelude to any teaching session.

5. The goals should be sufficient without being overwhelming

Successful teaching must include an element of challenge. Just as in the first commandment the teacher needs to feel that there is a real purpose in the teaching so the learner too needs to be stimulated without feeling overwhelmed. This is obvious but not that easy to achieve. Thorough prior assessment is essential if the teacher is to get this pitched at the right level.

6. The language should be clear and have meaning for the learner

Communication should be kept simple, convincing and familiar. This requires considerable preparation and thought. Quite often professional people use jargon as convenient shorthand and when really pressed for a definition in simple language are somewhat lost for a reply. It is also important that common words are used which have a shared meaning for both the teacher and the learner.

7. Teaching begins with what is familiar before moving to what is unfamiliar

The relationship between the teacher and the learner is important here. If a warm, relaxed and trustful atmosphere can be established in which people feel accepted this will enable them to assimilate new material more readily. Conversely, someone who is flooded with unfamiliar material will need to defend himself from the resultant anxiety that this induces, and learning will be minimised. If the teacher begins by sharing something familiar this will promote a feeling of mastery and confidence in the learner. Considerations of this kind are of special importance when people are under stress through pain and/or anxiety.

8. There should be variety in presentation to maintain interest and increase retention

Teaching is most effective when it is aimed at more than one of the senses. A very gifted speaker may enthral their audience for an hour or more but a more typical attention span would be between 7 and 10 minutes. Visual images are retained more easily than auditory ones. Active participatory learning in which both mind and body are involved tends to make an even greater impression. Learning in groups often provides greater stimulation and motivation than isolated learning.

9. Learning should be clearly structured to aid assimilation

Because a person's concentration span is limited much of the information received is not registered. Very often key points are selected and the rest discarded. The teacher must bear this in mind, presenting crucial material in a way which alerts the listener to its importance and offers continual signposts to these key points. Presentation should be structured in such a way that it offers guidance about what must be remembered, and what, although of interest and relevance is less important. Phrases like 'if you only remember one thing . . .' or 'the really crucial point is . . .' highlight clearly what is central and distinguish it from the peripheral and optional. It is important to time the message at the point when you are certain that you have fully engaged the hearers, e.g. when they are relatively fresh and wide awake.

10. Ways of evaluating outcomes should be devised before the teaching programme begins

One of the chief ways by which learners feel rewarded is through the recognition of their achievements. Whenever possible, people should be provided with feedback on their performance. This can be done by recording the goals which have been set and the progress which has been made towards them.

Learning will always result in some change occurring. This may consist of new ways of thinking, feeling or behaving, or any combination of these three. For example, a new knowledge of the resources which are available will change the way in which an issue is perceived and, in turn, both the feelings which relate to it and the actions which are taken in response to it. It is the task of the teacher to identify these changes and link them clearly to the learning which has taken place. This will provide the motivation needed to fuel enthusiasm for further work.

Exercise

Individually

- Identify a recent contact with service users where you were engaged in using teaching skills.
- Using the ten commandments as a checklist, see how many of them you kept in this instance.
- Examine those which were not kept and ask yourself whether their observation would have helped (i) the learner; (ii) yourself.

In groups

Share your review with other workers in order to:

- identify any common strengths and difficulties;
- decide whether these indicate that there are any training needs within the group to be addressed.

Educational skills in practice

Common educational situations that community practitioners meet include:

- health promotion with the general public;
- health education for the public;
- sharing skills with other carers, both lay and professional;
- sharing knowledge within one's own profession.

The purpose of this section is to draw attention to issues which will assist in preparation and presentation, rather than to teach how to be a teacher.

An educational session needs careful planning if it is to achieve its purpose of imparting knowledge and increasing understanding. Preparation needs to be thorough if the ten commandments of teaching are to be achieved.

Information gathering

When approached about or suggesting a session the following points are essential background:

When will the session be held?

Check that:

- The date and day of the week mentioned match.
- The start and finish times of your input are known, and whether this includes questions.

If you intend to use equipment it helps to know when you will have time for on-site preparation, such as loading slides and checking how equipment is controlled, or arranging exhibits.

These points are important if you are not the start of the event. Sometimes there is a business meeting or other speakers before you. You need to know whether you will have to arrive early or negotiate some time for this. It may affect your final choice of presentation. If a synopsis is required for publication of proceedings the date for submission also needs to be known.

Where will it take place?

Apart from the precise venue, with the address and directions on how to find it and the location of the room in the building, its size and what facilities are available need to be known. If you intend to show slides, a check on whether the venue has blackout facilities and a suitably sited power point is essential, apart from whether a screen and projector will be provided or you will need to take your own. If projection facilities are being provided check whether they will be front or back projection.

Always check who will provide any visual aids or other equipment you may need, and who will be ensuring that it is there in working order.

What is the topic required?

Sometimes community practitioners are approached to talk about their work in very general terms. It may require some suggestions or exploration of the topic to determine the information being sought within the context of the request.

Why is the session being held?

Is it part of a series, a continuation of a theme, to meet Health and Safety requirements, a part of a health fair or to share knowledge with other professionals? Has there been previous input on the subject? If so, is it a refresher session or an extension of knowledge?

The response to these questions helps determine the level of learning and possible content, as well as indicating the aim of the session.

Who will be the audience?

You need to know:

- Their background, e.g. professional or lay.
- Age range, as this indicates the life experience on which to build and helps decide how you might hold interest and make your audience feel involved.
- Previous experience related to the topic so that an appropriate starting level can be chosen.
- The anticipated number attending.

For some topics, such as practical skills teaching, there is a limit how many people can be taught at one time. This may be further affected by the space and facilities available. The number in the audience may also determine the presentation style or the teaching aids used. If you will require a person to use as a demonstration model, or a knowledgeable assistant, these needs should be discussed at this point, so that you can ensure who will be responsible for finding these people. You may need to meet them beforehand or be in touch about their input.

The other 'who' to clarify is the organiser or contact, with address and phone or fax number for any queries or needs which arise between the initial contact and your presentation.

Money

Perhaps this should come first! It is important that any fee and expenses are clarified at the initial contact so that the organiser can budget adequately. When discussing expenses, the costs of any special materials, such as handouts or non-reusable materials that might be wanted for practical skills acquisition, are costed. Clarification of travel and any other subsistence costs may also be required.

If you are organising the session there may be hire charges for the venue and for equipment, e.g. projectors, videos, which should be included in the budget.

More embarrassment and misunderstandings occur if the finances are not discussed and clarified at this early stage than those that might be felt by introducing finance in this business discussion.

How

Preparing the session

1. You as *teacher* need to decide what it is you want to achieve – the aim, goal or purpose of the session.
2. Decide what you want the *students* to be able to do by the end of the session – the objectives of the session. These will be testable as they use words like 'identify', and may have conditions attached such as 'without reference to notes', and a standard, e.g. 'four out of five samples'.
3. What shall be included? We all have a wealth of information, but if you think what:

- must
- should
- could

the students know, to be able to meet the objectives, it helps sort the material into the essential and non-essential, as well as clarifying the objectives.
4. Having decided the information that you intend to include, check reference material so that you have the latest information, or ensure that practical technique is well rehearsed and the theory behind it is at your fingertips.

Designing the session

Whatever the activities in the session a useful basic plan is:

Introduction
Clarify why you and they are there (the purpose, your aims),

indicate what you intend to do, and what they will be able to do at the end of the session. (Tell them what you are going to tell them.)

Main content or primary development of the topic
This should be logically sequenced in small progressive steps. (Tell them.)

Consolidation of information presented
This may be through examples or through some 'testing' and correcting, or various student-based activities.

Recapitulation or summary
This usually has key points which were your 'musts' when deciding what to include. (Tell them what you have told them.)

If you are taking a long session it may be appropriate to break it into sections following this plan. This not only helps the learner to absorb information but assists in providing a variety of activities. It also enables you to check learning of the different sections before moving on to the next in your presentation.

There are several ways of organising your notes for your session. Which method you choose will depend on the topic and your own personal preference.

Essay style
Here the section headings are used with 'paragraphs' subheaded by the activity when appropriate. It is advisable to leave gaps between the sections, and to have a margin to prompt the use of any teaching aids, such as change of slide or acetate on an overhead projector.

Columnar
Two or three columns are used with the teacher activity and key notes in one column, the student activity alongside in the second column, and teaching aids or equipment required listed in a third column.

Key words
Where there is a lot of demonstration, and material is very familiar, or lots of visual aids are being used, these may be adequate.

Two colour or highlighted
These are similar, but less detailed than essay, but have key words highlighted. This system is useful if small cards are being used.

Presenting a session – practical considerations

The room

Arrange the seating so that everyone can see, hear and actively participate. It may be necessary to rearrange the room or the audience if you are following on some other person, so it is appropriate for your activities.

As far as possible make sure the ventilation and heating are adequate, and external noise is minimised.

The students

Ensure that there is active participation. This may vary from ascertaining that everyone is still interested and awake to having everyone on the move or making something.

Involve as many of the students' senses as possible. Some learn by listening, others by seeing and some by doing.

Make sure all the students have understood each point before moving on to the next.

Organise the learning so that mistakes are minimised. Help students to understand where they have gone wrong if mistakes are made without putting down individuals before others.

Give approval for achievement and effort, and praise for success.

The teacher

Be well prepared with all equipment to hand and in order.

However nervous you feel, smile and look friendly, and show enthusiasm. Smiles and enthusiasm are infectious and create a receptive atmosphere.

Give guidance at the start on whether notes will need to be taken or handouts will be given. If you are dictating facts remember that people write at very variable rates, so state clearly and slowly in short phrases, and repeat each before going on to the next. If necessary, read the complete section through again at the end.

Let the students know before you start if they can ask questions at any time, or if you will be answering them at the end.

Speak in a language the students understand, explaining any technical terms or jargon you introduce.

If you have an accent that is pronounced and different from that of those you are speaking to, start slowly so that the audience can 'tune in', and avoid your local colloquialisms.

Beware of the 'ums' and 'ers'.

Avoid mannerisms, e.g. jiggling keys in your pocket, pulling your ear. They can be very distracting.

Make sure your material is relevant to the students' daily lives and experiences, as well as your aims.

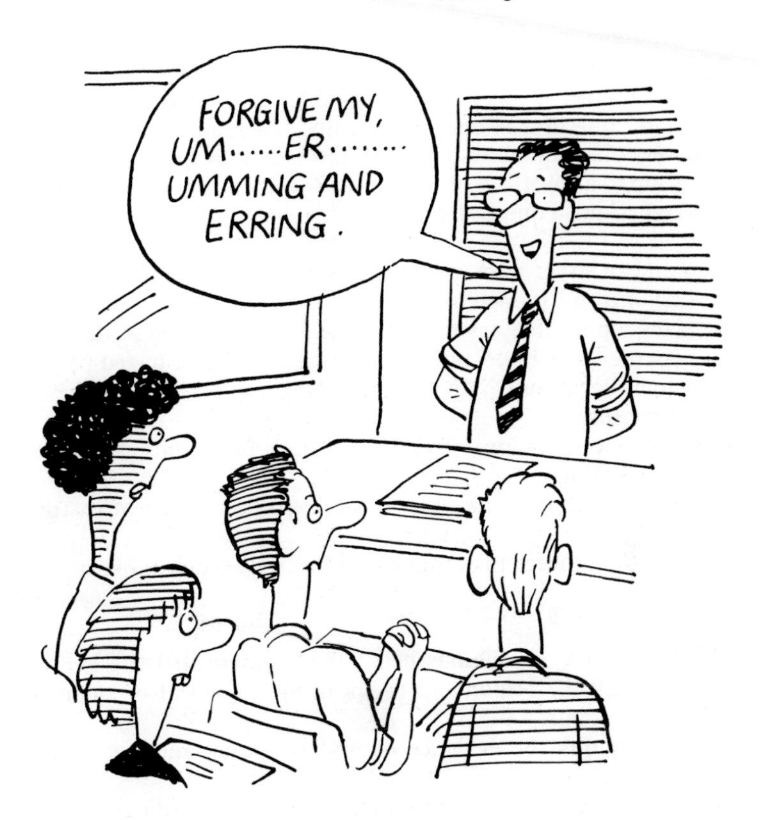

Use a variety of methods, e.g. talk, demonstration, video, role play, discussion, experiential, library research, computer program.

Make allowances for individual differences – we all learn at different rates and have different background experiences. Some people are extrovert, whilst others prefer to merge into the group. Be sensitive of these differences when involving students.

Questions

There are different reasons you may ask questions of your audience. These could be to:

- test knowledge;
- arouse curiosity;
- activate the class or an individual;
- gauge opinion;

- encourage expression;
- recapitulate.

A good question is one that is fully understood by the class, is unambiguous, stimulates thought and is within the capabilities of the group to answer.

When asking a question remember:

- You can either pose, pause then pounce, or name an individual first or throw it open to all.
- If it is applicable, try to match the question to the student. This is particularly important with a mixed ability or mixed previous knowledge group. You want the student to be able to achieve by answering.
- That the question should be clear, brief but explicit and unambiguous.
- To give the students time to think, so do not repeat it straight away.
- That one correct answer does not mean everyone knows.

When questions are answered:

- Make sure everyone has heard the response. If there is doubt, either ask the respondent to speak up, or repeat or summarise the key points.
- There should be evidence of understanding and not just rote response.
- Praise correct answers and do not condemn or ridicule wrong or poor answers. Use these as a basis for your next question.

When answering questions yourself:

- If it is relevant you can hand it back to the class to answer if it will reinforce their learning and stimulate discussion.
- If it is irrelevant answer briefly and move on.
- If you do not know the answer be honest and say so.
- If you say you will find out and let the students know, stay with your bargain and make sure you do, otherwise eventually your sins will find you out!

Teaching a skill

A useful sequence for teaching a skill within the lesson framework is:

1. Give the aim, and place it in context.

2. Demonstrate at normal speed, where possible repeating several times, and if necessary at different angles.
3. *Either:* break the action down into stages, *or* different body positions, explaining any key points with the reasons or repeat slowly, emphasising and verbalising key points.
4. Ask students to describe the action and key points.
5. Discuss safety factors.
6. Students' practise. They will only learn by doing. It may be necessary to break the task into stages. Correct mistakes early – it is difficult to erase bad habits.
As tutor:
- comment on accuracy, style, speed, quality, safety;
- do not give work beyond the mental and physical capacity;
- make sure the practice exercise does not require new skills over and above those demonstrated and taught;
- give confidence by praising and not blaming, seeing the right, stimulating to try again rather than harassing, and be sympathetic and encouraging;
- watch for boredom or fatique;
- encourage students to think through what they are doing and why.

7. Summarise the key points and point out that practice, with a knowledgeable commentator, makes perfect.

Visual aids

Visual aids are many and are intended to clarify points, provide information or to stimulate thought and discussion. They include:

- acetates for overhead projectors;
- blackboard, white board;
- flip chart;
- slides;
- video;
- demonstration models;
- samples;
- handouts.

With all check that:

- they are clear and can be readily seen by all the group;
- they are really applicable and appropriate to your session content;

- you are familiar with the material you are showing and with any apparatus, e.g. projectors, video playback, used with it
- if the material is the lynchpin of your session and has mechanical or electrical input, that you have either essential spare parts available or an alternative presentation method to hand if all else fails.

When preparing acetates, slides and flip charts remember:

- Projectors come with differently shaped and sized apertures, particularly overhead projectors. Keep to the central area of your acetate, and ensure the subject of your slide is central when taking the photograph.
- Do not overcrowd information. Keep layout simple and clear.
- To think about the use of colour. Sometimes it can be helpful and others confusing.
- If you are having slides made of text, white on a blue background is easier on the eye than black on white. Use horizontal format, as this projects better in a large hall and allows for the screen shape. At some conferences the organisers specify horizontal format for this reason.

When using videos, film (or audiotape) make sure that you have viewed them and selected the appropriate section in advance. If you intend to show an extract make sure that the tape is ready at the appropriate point beforehand. If playing more than one extract, note on the counter where you need to fast-forward to so that you are not searching during your session.

Conclusion

Finally, allow yourself plenty of time to arrive at the venue – Murphy's Law says that speakers and lecturers will always be prone to a delay. Give yourself time to check through your material, make yourself familiar with the venue, and to make yourself comfortable before you start.

Exercises

1. Individually respond then compare your answers with others and discuss any similarities or differences.

- What helps you to learn and remember?
- What 'turns you off' from learning?

2. Note down good learning experiences you can recall and bad ones. Try to analyse why these were so. Are there any points that you can learn from for your own presentations?
3. Pick a topic you feel comfortable with and are often having to teach. Using what you have learnt from this chapter, prepare a session outline.

Supervision

Introduction

This section can only offer a very brief introduction to supervision. It is a skilled process and training for it is essential. It is worth investigating the support and training available to you if you are approached to undertake professional supervision. It cannot be assumed that it will be available.

Exercise

Before reading this section, write down all your immediate reactions to the word 'supervisor'. If you are part of a training group share your reactions with each other. Think about and, if in a group, discuss these reactions. How will they influence your attitude to being supervised and your attitude to supervising?

The need for supervision

Helpers, however well trained, work with people under stress, often in environments which are frustrating and where resources are limited. In an investigation into social practitioners' experience of stress, social practitioners were quick to recognise signs of stress in other colleagues, if not quite so readily in themselves (King 1991). The majority of those interviewed included supervision in the factors which would help minimise stress.

Many helpers, in reality, do not find it easy accepting supervision when it is offered. Hawkins and Shohet (1989) quote Claxton's (1984) four beliefs that get in the way of adult learning. They are:

1. I must be competent.
2. I must be in control.
3. I must be consistent.
4. I must be comfortable.

They make the point that these beliefs are capable of sabotaging exploration. If they go unchallenged they may actually become intensified as supervisee becomes supervisor and then a supervisor of supervisors. 'Trainers have to model not being super competent in control experts who are still open to and needing to learn and who are also open about their vulnerability' (Claxton 1984, page 81).

For many helpers supervision sessions are few and far between. They may be given low priority and become one of the first things to go in a supervisor's crowded schedule. Often they are sacrificed to the 'greater' needs of service users or managers.

The new language of the market has entered the helping professions. This emphasises concepts like consumerism, choice and quality control. This may well have a positive energising effect but will be self defeating if the producers of aspects of care are not properly supervised and maintained.

There is a slowly growing recognition of the need for supervision as a tool of management, training and support. It is for this reason that most practitioners will become trainers and supervisors not that long after completing training.

The supervisor's accountability

For me the word 'supervision' conjure up a picture of the factory floor and quality control relating to production of goods. It seemed a somewhat inappropriate description for many of the tasks commonly associated with supervision. The *Shorter Oxford Dictionary*'s definition was 'the action or function of supervising, oversight and superintendance' which did little to banish this image. Indeed there is a very real sense in which supervision is about monitoring outputs. The supervisor will be accountable to three different and sometimes conflicting groups. These are:

1. The supervisor's employing agency

This agency will expect from the supervisor:

- The maintenance of acceptable professional standards.
- The proper and efficient use of resources, e.g. time, equipment.
- The teaching of new skills demanded because of professional/organisational change.
- That he or she will ensure that the supervisee has an understanding of and sufficient identification with the goals of the agency.

- That the supervisee is enabled to liaise with other helping agencies to provide an integrated service.

2. *The service users*

They have a right to expect that supervisors will ensure that:

- The supervisee has the appropriate knowledge and skills to perform the professional task.
- Their rights will be protected in relation to confidentiality, self determination, choice and information and access to resources and grievance procedures.
- The supervisee will conduct the relationship in an ethical and competent manner.
- The worker is able to communicate and cooperate with other helping agencies to produce a maximised integrated service.

3. *The supervisee*

In order to meet the needs of their supervisees a supervisor should be able to:

- Establish a relationship with the supervisee which is open and reliable.
- Delineate the boundaries of the supervisory contract (the where, when, what, why, who and how of the arrangement).
- Demonstrate an appropriate level of knowledge and skills needed to facilitate professional and personal development.
- Provide a role model which is orientated to growth and creativity rather than conformity and rigidity.

It is not always easy to reconcile all these expectations. The task of the supervisor can be seen, rightly, as challenging and demanding.

Exercise

Individually or in groups examine each of these three sources of expectations, then:

- decide whether you accept the content under each heading;
- identify any changes that you would like to make either by making additions or amendments.

The qualities of the supervisor

The idea that all supervisors are professional paragons is, of course, absurd. The gap between the supervisor and the supervisee in terms of knowledge and experience may be quite small. In peer supervision it may be non-existent. What separates the one from the other is the availability of the supervisor to be placed at the disposal of the supervisee as an enabling and empowering agent.

What supervisors should offer, as well as time, space and attention are:

- A proper and detailed knowledge of the tasks of the supervisee.
- A clear understanding of the relationship between the agency and the other community resources and of their communication networks.
- A commitment to the provision of a quality service to agency users.
- An understanding of the supervisory process and the ability to make it a reality.
- A belief and commitment to the importance of personal growth as an essential component of professional development.

Exercise

In groups of three, each person will take it in turns to play the part of supervisor, supervisee and observer.

The supervisee will bring an incident from their recent work about which they have unresolved feelings and discuss this with the supervisor for 7 to 10 minutes.

The supervisor will try to ensure that he or she:

- has heard the entire story;
- has understood why the supervisee is concerned;
- has explored the possible professional responses to the incident discussed.

The observer will feed back to:

- the supervisee on his/her ability to accept and use the supervisor's interventions;
- the supervisor on his/her ability to establish rapport, understand the problem and respond creatively to it.

The delivery of supervision

Supervision takes place within a certain setting. It is part of a distinct process and will address particular issues. Each of these will be briefly considered here.

The setting

The provision of supervision within the training agency is a possible way of valuing and supporting practitioners. The way in which supervisory sessions are organised will either deny or confirm this possibility. Basically it is hard to uphold high standards of concern and respect for clients if supervisors do not model these qualities in relation to their supervisees.

This concern and respect should be demonstrated in the protection of the supervisory session against encroachments and interruptions. The actual session should afford privacy and a reasonable level of physical comfort so that distractions are minimised.

The process

The basic supervisory process is identical with that of any other planned intervention. It will consist of an assessment, a contract and a programme. This programme will be monitored and, when completed, evaluated. New goals may then be negotiated, based upon an updated appraisal.

Important decisions have to be made in relation to this process. They relate to the method of assessment, the nature of the contract and the implementation of the programme. They will often be concerned with basic details such as what will be recorded, by whom and who will have access to the material.

The establishment of a clear operational framework acts as a protection to both supervisor and supervisee in what is a very sensitive area of work. The strength of the boundaries will determine the nature of the containment offered. This containment in turn will determine the depth and scope of the work which can be undertaken.

The content

The content of supervisory sessions is a matter of negotiation. Both supervisors and supervisees will have expectations and needs. Hawkins and Shohet (1989) remind us of Heron's (1975) six categories of intervention. These consists of the following types:

Prescriptive
This would involve the supervisor in giving clear guidelines to the supervisee. The tone is directive and authoritative.

Informative
This concerns the giving of information or instruction. It is a teaching mode.

Confrontative
This offers challenge to the supervisee yet is more demanding in nature, asking for further exploration and consideration.

Cathartic
This allows the supervisee to let off steam and express some of the pent-up feelings, the suppression of which may be absorbing some of the valuable problem-solving energy.

Catalytic
In this type of intervention the supervisee enables the worker to explore, make corrections and develop their own unique style of helping rooted in sound practice.

Supportive
Here the supervisor is concerned to support, confirm and uphold the supervisee. It is what every one says they want but helpers may still find it harder to receive than to give because of fear of dependence.

These categories offer a very useful method of analysis. Good supervision will probably consist of a range of these interventions. Very heavy dependence on one type is probably a danger sign.

Exercise

In groups of three, taking it in turns to be supervisor, supervisee and observer:

- The supervisee will explore a current professional task of real importance for 7 to 10 minutes.
- The supervisor will help the exploration, keeping in mind the needs of the service users and the demands of the agency as well as the immediate concerns of the supervisee.
- The observer will use Heron's six categories as a check list and feedback to the supervisor how these were employed by

the supervisor during the session. Any unclear interventions will be discussed.

- The supervisee and the supervisor will share their experience of the session, particularly noting any difference in perception, and exploring reasons for these.

References

Claxton, G. (1984) *Live and Learn.* London: Harper and Row.

Coutts, L. C. and Hardy, L. K. (1985) *Teaching for Health – the Nurse as Health Educator.* Edinburgh: Churchill Livingstone.

Ewles, L. and Simnett, I. (1980) *Promoting Health – a Practical Guide to Health Education.*

Education for Health – a Manual on Health Education in Primary Health Care. Geneva: World Health Organisation (1988).

Hawkins, P. and Shohet, R. (1989) *Supervision in the Helping Professions.* Milton Keynes: Open University Press.

Heron, J. (1975) Six Category Interventional Analysis. Guildford, Surrey: University of Surrey Human Potential Research Project.

King, J. (1991) Taking the strain, *Community Care,* issue no. 886, 24 October.

Additional reading

Curzon, L. C. (1980) *Teaching in Further Education* (2nd edn). London: Cassell.

Rogers, J. (1977) *Adults Learning* (2nd edn). Milton Keynes: Open University Press.

Chapter 12

Concluding exercises – cases to resolve

Ann Compton

Do these individually then get together with others and compare solutions, and your reasons? There is no one answer, and those reached will depend upon your local resources and the nature of the group members' backgrounds.

It is helpful to list for each individual, using the 'problem, resources, constraints' columns and then to look at the common concerns to decide where to start, and with what.

Remember to look at work, education, health, social and voluntary aspects, and to take account of social and cultural backgrounds.

1. Mrs Smith, 36, has just entered a remission after an acute phase of multiple sclerosis, leaving her with increased spasticity of both legs and occasional urinary incontinence. She is now able to walk about 5 yards at a time with some difficulty using a frame. Her arms and sight seem normal, but she does get fatigued quickly. She is mentally alert, and a sensible and practical person, who has always been cheerful and friendly. She worked as a checkout assistant in a big grocery chain, taking maternity leave for John, until Jane was due, putting her early signs of leg pains and stumbling down to her first pregnancy, and fatigue to coping with her first baby.

Mr Smith, 37, after a year's unemployment has obtained work as a general storeman at the supermarket 1 mile away in the opposite direction from the local school. He had previously been senior storeman for a large factory which closed in a major company reorganisation. This involves him at present being on early and late shifts alternately with once a month Saturday working. He is very caring and supportive of his wife and family, who are John, 8, Jane, 5, and Jimmy, just 3. They live in a three-bedroomed mid-terrace council house with upstairs bath and WC, with a lounge-diner and kitchen downstairs. Their relatives, her arthritic mother and divorced sister's family of 10-year-old and 8-year-old girls, live 6 miles away, but can offer little practical help during the week.

Mr Smith has a younger brother in the army posted abroad living in married quarters with his wife and new baby.

Indicate the services and provisions that might be made for the family, and note the professionals, together with their input, who might be involved. Note the liaison required between those you decide will be assisting the family.

2. A Hindu, who is the head of his family, had a stroke 6 weeks ago affecting his right side. He has some shoulder, hip and knee movement, but no other arm or hand movement nor ankle movement. He is able to stand with support.

He has been in Britain for about 19 years, and it is known that he only uses English for his business needs, since he lives and socialises within his own national community. His wife has very limited English but his children, five sons and three daughters, all had some or all of their schooling in Britain.

He lives in a flat above one of his three shops, of which two are run by his oldest sons working long hours. He was still running his original shop himself with his two younger sons working alongside him and their brothers.

He is well cared for by his family but has not made any attempt to try to help himself. He has a Hindi-speaking GP who mentions that his speech is hesitant. There is a Hindi-speaking community practitioner who is used by the local medical professional staff, who are mostly female.

Consider how you might be able to assist.

3. This referral has been received by the physiotherapist from her GP: 'Mrs Fay, age 62, of Laneside, Old Street, Layby. tel: Layby 221. Osteoarthritic knees with loss of mobility, pain and joint swelling. Lives alone with dog on smallholding away from village. Recently widowed. Out Weds. – village lunch club/WI.'

Drugs and tubigrip prescribed are noted, together with 'considering orthopaedic referral, your assessment awaited'.

The physiotherapist, when at the surgery, finds that Mr Fay died suddenly about 18 months ago from a heart attack shortly after winning a national championship for best of breed with his goats, which he and his wife had kept for years. Mrs Fay still had a few goats, though she had cut down on livestock and kept only the champion breeding blood and a few hens. She still sold some goat's milk and its products, and some free range eggs. She had coped well with her bereavement, thanks to her village friends.

Note the implications of 'loss of mobility' to Mrs Fay. Whose services is she likely to need, other than the physiotherapist's advice?

4. The much wanted son and newly born second child of a young executive and his wife in their late thirties has Down's syndrome. He is now being taken home, but the parents have not yet said anything to their friends or neighbours, although their immediate families know. Their 4½-year-old daughter is aware Mummy and Daddy are upset, and has been told by them and her grandparents, who came to stay, that her baby brother, whom she saw at the hospital, is going to be slower growing up than she was herself. She was told to tell her friends at her private nursery school that her new brother was not very well, and she heard her grandmother say this to her teacher, whom she likes very much.

What can be done to help this family (a) now, (b) over the next 2 years and (c) as the boy grows up?

Index